Toward Precision Medicine

Building a Knowledge Network for Biomedical Research
and a New Taxonomy of Disease

Committee on A Framework for Developing a
New Taxonomy of Disease

Board on Life Sciences

Division on Earth and Life Studies

NATIONAL RESEARCH COUNCIL
OF THE NATIONAL ACADEMIES

THE NATIONAL ACADEMIES PRESS
Washington, D.C.
www.nap.edu

THE NATIONAL ACADEMIES PRESS   500 Fifth Street NW   Washington, DC 20001

NOTICE: The project that is the subject of this report was approved by the Governing Board of the National Research Council, whose members are drawn from the councils of the National Academy of Sciences, the National Academy of Engineering, and the Institute of Medicine. The members of the Committee responsible for the report were chosen for their special competences and with regard for appropriate balance.

This study was supported by Contract/Grant No. N01-0D-4-2139 between the National Academy of Sciences and the National Institutes of Health. Any opinions, findings, conclusions, or recommendations expressed in this publication are those of the author(s) and do not necessarily reflect the views of the organizations or agencies that provided support for the project.

International Standard Book Number-13:   978-0-309-22222-8
International Standard Book Number-10:   0-309-22222-2
Library of Congress Control Number: 2011943146

Additional copies of this report are available from the National Academies Press, 500 Fifth Street, N.W., Lockbox 285, Washington, DC 20055; (800) 624-6242 or (202) 334-3313 (in the Washington metropolitan area); Internet, http://www.nap.edu

Cover art: Nicolle Rager Fuller, Sayo-Art LLC
Photo: © Graham Bell/Corbis

THE NATIONAL ACADEMIES
Advisers to the Nation on Science, Engineering, and Medicine

The **National Academy of Sciences** is a private, nonprofit, self-perpetuating society of distinguished scholars engaged in scientific and engineering research, dedicated to the furtherance of science and technology and to their use for the general welfare. Upon the authority of the charter granted to it by the Congress in 1863, the Academy has a mandate that requires it to advise the federal government on scientific and technical matters. Dr. Ralph J. Cicerone is president of the National Academy of Sciences.

The **National Academy of Engineering** was established in 1964, under the charter of the National Academy of Sciences, as a parallel organization of outstanding engineers. It is autonomous in its administration and in the selection of its members, sharing with the National Academy of Sciences the responsibility for advising the federal government. The National Academy of Engineering also sponsors engineering programs aimed at meeting national needs, encourages education and research, and recognizes the superior achievements of engineers. Dr. Charles M. Vest is president of the National Academy of Engineering.

The **Institute of Medicine** was established in 1970 by the National Academy of Sciences to secure the services of eminent members of appropriate professions in the examination of policy matters pertaining to the health of the public. The Institute acts under the responsibility given to the National Academy of Sciences by its congressional charter to be an adviser to the federal government and, upon its own initiative, to identify issues of medical care, research, and education. Dr. Harvey V. Fineberg is president of the Institute of Medicine.

The **National Research Council** was organized by the National Academy of Sciences in 1916 to associate the broad community of science and technology with the Academy's purposes of furthering knowledge and advising the federal government. Functioning in accordance with general policies determined by the Academy, the Council has become the principal operating agency of both the National Academy of Sciences and the National Academy of Engineering in providing services to the government, the public, and the scientific and engineering communities. The Council is administered jointly by both Academies and the Institute of Medicine. Dr. Ralph J. Cicerone and Dr. Charles M. Vest are chair and vice chair, respectively, of the National Research Council.

www.national-academies.org

BOARD ON LIFE SCIENCES

Acknowledgments

This report has been reviewed in draft form by individuals chosen for their diverse perspectives and technical expertise in accordance with procedures approved by the National Research Council's Report Review Committee. The purpose of this independent review is to provide candid and critical comments that will assist the institution in making its published report as sound as possible and to ensure that the report meets institutional standards of objectivity, evidence, and responsiveness to the study charge. The review comments and draft manuscript remain confidential to protect the integrity of the deliberative process.

We thank the following individuals for their review of this report:

- **Leslie Biesecker,** *National Institutes of Health*
- **Martin J. Blaser,** *New York University Langone Medical Center*
- **Wylie Burke,** *University of Washington*
- **Christopher G. Chute,** *University of Minnesota and Mayo Clinic*
- **Sean Eddy,** *Howard Hughes Medical Institute Janelia Farm Research*
- **Elaine Jaffe,** *National Cancer Institute*
- **Brian J. Kelly,** *Aetna*
- **Chaitan Khosla,** *Stanford University*
- **Daniel R. Masys,** *University of Washington*
- **Stephen M. Schwartz,** *University of Washington*

Although the reviewers listed above have provided many constructive comments and suggestions, they were not asked to endorse the conclusions or recommendations, nor did they see the final draft of the report before its release. The review of the report was overseen by **Dennis Ausiello,** *Harvard Medical School, Massachusetts General Hospital and Partners Healthcare,* and

Queta Bond, *Burroughs Wellcome Fund.* Appointed by the National Research Council, they were responsible for making certain that an independent examination of this report was carried out in accordance with institutional procedures and that all review comments were carefully considered. Responsibility for the final content of the report rests entirely with the authoring committee and the institution.

We thank Dr. Theresa O'Brien, Director of Research Strategy and Special Projects, UCSF School of Medicine, for thoughtful suggestions and support to the Committee and NRC staff, throughout this study process. We thank Steve Olson for his writing and editorial assistance.

We are grateful to those who attended and participated in the workshop "Toward a New Taxonomy of Disease," held March 1 and 2, 2011 (Appendix C) and those who discussed data sharing with the Committee during the course of this study. These individuals, named below, were generous with their time, expertise, and ideas, and their insights were helpful to the Committee's work:

- **Charles Baum**, *Vice President of Global R&D, Pfizer*
- **Leslie Biesecker**, *Chief & Senior Investigator, Genetic Disease Research Branch, NHGRI*
- **Martin Blaser**, *Frederick H. King Professor of Internal Medicine and Chairman of the Department of Medicine, NYU School of Medicine*
- **John Brownstein**, *Instructor, Harvard Medical School*
- **Atul Butte**, *Chief and Assistant Professor, Division of Systems Medicine, Department of Pediatrics, Stanford*
- **Lewis Cantley**, *Chief, Division of Signal Transduction, Harvard Medical School*
- **Alta Charo**, *Professor of Law and Bioethics, University of Wisconsin Law School*
- **Christopher G. Chute**, *Professor of Medical Informatics, Mayo Clinic College of Medicine*
- **Andrew Conrad**, *Chief Scientific Officer, LabCorp*
- **Elissa Epel**, *Associate Professor in Residence, Department of Psychiatry at University of California, San Francisco*
- **Kathy Giusti**, *Founder and Chief Executive Officer, Multiple Myeloma Research Foundation (MMRF)*
- **John Glaser**, *Chief Executive Officer, Health Services Business Unit, Siemens Health Services*
- **Corey Goodman**, *Managing Director and Co-Founder, venBio*
- **Brian J. Kelly**, *Head of Informatics and Strategic Alignment, Aetna*
- **Debra Lappin**, *President, Council for American Medical Innovation*
- **Jason Lieb**, *Professor, Department of Biology, University of North Carolina at Chapel Hill*
- **Klaus Lindpaintner**, *Vice President of R&D, Strategic Diagnostics Inc.*

- **Jon Lorsch,** *Professor of Biophysics and Biophysical Chemistry, Johns Hopkins University, School of Medicine*
- **Daniel Masys,** *Chair of the Department of Biomedical Informatics, Vanderbilt University Medical Center*
- **William Pao,** *Director, Personalized Cancer Medicine at the Vanderbilt-Ingram Cancer Center*
- **Erin Ramos,** *Epidemiologist, National Human Genome Research Institute*
- **Neil Risch,** *Institute for Human Genetics, University of California, San Francisco*
- **Catherine Schaefer,** *Kaiser Permanente Northern California Division of Research*
- **Ingrid Scheffer,** *Professor of Paediatric Neurology Research, University of Melbourne*
- **Sanford Schwartz,** *Professor of Medicine, Health Care Management, and Economics, University of Pennsylvania*
- **Janet Woodcock,** *Director, Center for Drug Evaluation and Research at the U.S. Food and Drug Administration*
- **Helmut Zarbl,** *University of Medicine and Dentistry of New Jersey-Robert Wood Johnson Medical School, Environmental & Occupational Medicine, Rutgers University*

Contents

BOXES

FIGURES

Summary

The Committee's charge was to explore the feasibility and need for "a New Taxonomy of human disease based on molecular biology" and to develop a potential framework for creating one. Clearly, the motivation for this study is the explosion of molecular data on humans, particularly those associated with individual patients, and the sense that there are large, as-yet-untapped opportunities to use these data to improve health outcomes. The Committee agreed with this perspective and, indeed, came to see the challenge of developing a New Taxonomy of Disease as just one element, albeit an important one, in a truly historic set of health-related challenges and opportunities associated with the rise of data-intensive biology and rapidly expanding knowledge of the mechanisms of fundamental biological processes. Hence, many of the implications of the Committee's findings and recommendations ramify far beyond the science of disease classification and have substantial implications for nearly all stakeholders in the vast enterprise of biomedical research and patient care.

Given the scope of the Committee's deliberations, it is appropriate to start this report by tracing the logical thread that unifies the Committee's major findings and recommendations and connects them to its statement of task. The Committee's charge highlights the importance of taxonomy in medicine and the potential opportunities to use molecular data to improve disease taxonomy and, thereby, health outcomes. Taxonomy is the practice and science of classification, typically considered in the context of biology (e.g., the Linnaean system for classifying living organisms). In medical practice, taxonomy often refers to the International Classification of Diseases (ICD), a system established more than 100 years ago that the World Health Organization uses to track disease incidence, physicians use as a basis for standardized diagnoses, and the health-care industry (specifically, clinicians, hospitals, and payers) uses to

1

determine reimbursement for care. Although the Committee was cognizant that any new-taxonomy initiative must serve the needs of the ICD and related classification systems, it concluded that this goal could best be met by rooting future improvements in disease classification in an "Information Commons" and "Knowledge Network" that would play many other roles, as well. The Committee envisions these data repositories as essential infrastructure, necessary both for creating the New Taxonomy and, more broadly, for integrating basic biological knowledge with medical histories and health outcomes of individual patients. The Committee believes that building this infrastructure—the Information Commons and Knowledge Network—is a grand challenge that, if met, would both modernize the ways in which biomedical research is conducted and, over time, lead to dramatically improved patient care (see Figure S-1).

The Committee envisions this ambitious program, which would play out on a time scale of decades rather than years, as proceeding through a blend of top-down and bottom-up activity. A major top-down component, initiated by public and private agencies that fund and regulate biomedical research, would be required to ensure that results of individual projects could be combined to

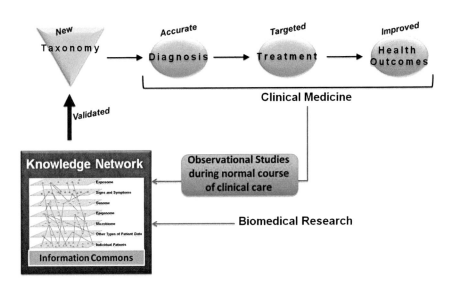

FIGURE S-1 Creation of a New Taxonomy first requires an "Information Commons" in which data on large populations of patients become broadly available for research use and a "Knowledge Network" that adds value to these data by highlighting their inter-connectedness and integrating them with evolving knowledge of fundamental biological processes.
SOURCE: Committee on A Framework for Developing a New Taxonomy of Disease.

create a broadly useful and accessible Information Commons and to establish guidelines for handling the innumerable social, ethical, and legal issues that will arise as data on individual patients become widely shared research resources. However, as is appropriate for a framework study, the Committee did not attempt to design the Information Commons, the Knowledge Network, or the New Taxonomy itself and would discourage funding agencies from over-specifying these entities in advance of initial efforts to create them. What is needed, in the Committee's view, is a creative period of bottom-up research activity, organized through pilot projects of increasing scope and scale, from which the Committee is confident best practices would emerge. Particularly given the size and diversity of the health-care enterprise, no one approach to gathering the data that will populate the Information Commons is likely to be appropriate for all contributors. As in any initiative of this complexity, what will be needed is the right level of coordination and encouragement of the many players who will need to cooperate to create the Information Commons and Knowledge Network and thereby develop a New Taxonomy. If coordination is too rigid, much-needed innovation and adaptation to local circumstances will be stifled, while if it is too lax, it will be impossible to integrate the data that are gathered into a whole whose value greatly exceeds that of the sum of its parts, an objective the Committee believes is achievable with effective central leadership.

CONCLUSIONS

The Committee hosted a two-day workshop that convened diverse experts in both basic and clinical disease biology to address the feasibility, need, scope, impact, and consequences of creating a "New Taxonomy of human diseases based on molecular biology". The information and opinions conveyed at the workshop informed and influenced an intensive series of Committee deliberations (in person and by teleconference) over a six-month period, which led to the following conclusions:

1. **A New Taxonomy will lead to better health care.** Because new information and concepts from biomedical research cannot be optimally incorporated into the disease taxonomy of today, opportunities to define diseases more precisely and to inform health-care decisions are being missed. Many disease subtypes with distinct molecular causes are still classified as one disease and, conversely, multiple different diseases share a common molecular cause. The failure to incorporate optimally new biological insights results in delayed adoption of new practice guidelines and wasteful health-care expenditures for treatments that are only effective in specific subgroups.

2. **The time is right to modernize disease taxonomy.** Dramatic advances in molecular biology have enabled rapid, comprehensive and

cost-efficient analysis of clinical samples, resulting in an explosion of disease-relevant data with the potential to dramatically alter disease classification. Fundamental discovery research is defining at the molecular level the processes that define and drive physiology. These developments, coupled with parallel advances in information technologies and electronic medical records, provide a transformative opportunity to create a new system to classify disease.

3. **A New Taxonomy should be developed.** A New Taxonomy that integrates multi-parameter molecular data with clinical data, environmental data, and health outcomes in a dynamic, iterative fashion, is feasible and should be developed. The Committee envisions a comprehensive disease taxonomy that brings the biomedical-research, public health, and health-care-delivery communities together around the related goals of advancing our understanding of disease pathogenesis and improving health. Such a New Taxonomy would

   - Describe and define diseases based on their intrinsic biology in addition to traditional physical "signs and symptoms."
   - Go beyond description and be directly linked to a deeper understanding of disease mechanisms, pathogenesis, and treatments.
   - Be highly dynamic, at least when used as a research tool, continuously incorporating newly emerging disease information.

4. **A Knowledge Network of Disease would Enable a New Taxonomy.** The informational infrastructure required to create a New Taxonomy with the characteristics described above overlaps with that required to modernize many other facets of biomedical research and patient care. This infrastructure requires an "Information Commons" in which data on large populations of patients become broadly available for research use and a "Knowledge Network" that adds value to these data by highlighting their inter-connectedness and integrating them with evolving knowledge of fundamental biological processes.

5. **New models for population-based research will enable development of the Knowledge Network and New Taxonomy.** Current population-based studies of disease are relatively inefficient and can generate conclusions that are not relevant to broader populations. Widespread incorporation of electronic medical records into the health-care system will make it possible to conduct such research at "point-of-care" in conjunction with the routine delivery of medical services. Moreover, only if the linked phenotypic data is acquired in the ordinary course of clinical care is it likely to be economically feasible to characterize a sufficient number of patients and ultimately to create a self-sustaining system (i.e., one in which the costs of gathering molecular data on individual patients can be medically justified in cost-benefit terms).

6. **Redirection of resources could facilitate development of the Knowledge Network of Disease.** The initiative to develop a New Taxonomy—and its underlying Information Commons and Knowledge Network—is a needed modernization of current approaches to integrating molecular, environmental, and phenotypic data, not an "add-on" to existing research programs. Enormous efforts are already underway to achieve many of the goals of this report. In the Committee's view, what is missing is a system-wide emphasis on shifting the large-scale acquisition of molecular data to point-of-care settings and the coordination required to ensure that the products of the research will coalesce into an Information Commons and Knowledge Network from which a New Taxonomy (and many other benefits) can be derived. In view of this conclusion, the Committee makes no recommendations about the resource requirements of the New Taxonomy initiative. Obviously, the process could be accelerated with new resources; however, the basic thrust of the Committee's recommendations could be pursued by redirection of resources already dedicated to increasing the medical utility of large-scale molecular datasets on individual patients.

RECOMMENDATIONS

To create a New Taxonomy and its underlying Information Commons and Knowledge Network, the Committee recommends the following:

1. **Conduct pilot studies that begin to populate the Information Commons with data.** Pilot observational studies should be conducted in the health-care setting to assess the feasibility of integrating molecular parameters with medical histories and health outcomes in the ordinary course of clinical care. These studies would address the practical and ethical challenges involved in creating, linking, and making broadly accessible the datasets that would underlie the New Taxonomy. Best practices defined by the pilot studies should then be expanded in scope and scale to produce an Information Commons and Knowledge Network that are adequately powered to support a New Taxonomy. As this process evolves, there should be ongoing assessment of the extent to which these new informational resources actually contribute to improved health outcomes and to more cost-effective delivery of health care.

2. **Integrate Data to Construct a Disease Knowledge Network.** As data from point-of-care pilot studies, linked to individual patients, begin to populate the Information Commons, substantial effort should go into integrating these data with the results of basic biomedical research

in order to create a dynamic, interactive Knowledge Network. This network, and the Information Commons itself, should leverage state-of-the-art information technology to provide multiple views of the data, as appropriate to the varying needs of different users (e.g., basic researchers, clinicians, outcomes researchers, payers).

3. **Initiate a process within an appropriate federal agency to assess the privacy issues associated with the research required to create the Information Commons.** Because these issues have been studied extensively, this process need not start from scratch. However, in practical terms, investigators who wish to participate in the pilot studies discussed above—and the Institutional Review Boards who must approve their human-subjects protocols—will need specific guidance on the range of informed-consent processes appropriate for these projects. Subject to the constraints of current law and prevailing ethical standards, the Committee encourages as much flexibility as possible in the guidance provided. As much as possible, on-the-ground experience in pilot projects carried out in diverse health-care settings, rather than top-down dictates, should govern the emergence of best practices in this sensitive area, whose handling will have a make-or-break influence on the entire Information Commons/Knowledge Network/New Taxonomy initiative. Inclusion in these deliberations of health-care providers, payers, and other stakeholders outside the academic community will be essential.

4. **Ensure data sharing.** Widespread data sharing is critical to the success of each stage of the process by which the Committee envisions creating a New Taxonomy. Most fundamentally, the molecular and phenotypic data on individual patients that populate the Information Commons must be broadly accessible so that a wide diversity of researchers can mine them for specific purposes and explore alternate ways of deriving Knowledge Networks and disease taxonomies from them. Current standards developed and adopted by federally sponsored genome projects have addressed some of these issues, but substantial barriers, particularly to the sharing of phenotypic and health-outcomes data on individual patients, remain. Data-sharing standards should be created that respect individual privacy concerns while enhancing the deposition of data into the Information Commons. Importantly, these standards should provide incentives that motivate data sharing over the establishment of proprietary databases for commercial intent. Resolving these impediments may require legislation and perhaps evolution in the public's expectations with regard to access and privacy of health-care data.

5. **Develop an efficient validation process to incorporate information from the Knowledge Network of Disease into a New Taxonomy.**

Insights into disease classification that emerge from the Information Commons and the derived Knowledge Network will require validation of their reproducibility and their utility for making clinically relevant distinctions (e.g., regarding prognosis or choice of treatment) before adoption into clinical use. A process should be established by which such information is validated for incorporation into a New Taxonomy to be used by physicians, patients, regulators, and payers. The speed and complexity with which such validated information emerges will undoubtedly accelerate and will require novel decision-support systems for use by all stakeholders.

6. **Incentivize partnerships.** The Committee envisions that a New Taxonomy incorporating molecular data could become self-sustaining by accelerating delivery of better health through more accurate diagnosis and more effective and cost-efficient treatments. However, to cover initial costs associated with collecting and integrating data for the Information Commons, incentives should be developed that encourage public–private partnerships involving government, drug developers, regulators, advocacy groups, and payers.

A major beneficiary of the proposed Knowledge Network of Disease and New Taxonomy would be what has been termed "precision medicine." The Committee is of the opinion that realizing the full promise of precision medicine, whose goal is to provide the best available care for each individual, requires that researchers and health-care providers have access to vary large sets of health and disease-related data linked to individual patients. These data are also critical for the development of the Information Commons, the Knowledge Network of Disease, and the development and validation of the New Taxonomy.

1

Introduction

THE CURRENT OPPORTUNITY

Biomedical research and the practice of medicine, separately and together, are reaching an inflection point: the capacity for description and for collecting data, is expanding dramatically, but the efficiency of compiling, organizing, manipulating these data—and extracting true understanding of fundamental biological processes, and insights into human health and disease, from them—has not kept pace. There are isolated examples of progress: research in certain diseases using genomics, proteomics, metabolomics, systems analyses, and other modern tools has begun to yield tangible medical advances, while some insightful clinical observations have spurred new hypotheses and laboratory efforts. In general, however, there is a growing shortfall: without better integration of information both within and between research and medicine, an increasing wealth of information is left unused.

As illustration, consider the following clinical scenarios;[1] in the first example, molecular understanding of disease has already begun to play an important role in informing treatment decisions, while in the second, it has not.

Patient 1 is consulting with her medical oncologist following breast cancer surgery. Twenty-five years ago, the patient's mother had breast cancer, when therapeutic options were few: hormonal suppression or broad-spectrum chemotherapy with significant side effects. Today, Patient 1's physician can suggest a precise regimen of therapeutic options tailored to the molecular characteristics of her cancer, drawn from among multiple therapies that together focus on her particular tumor markers. Moreover, the patient's relatives can undergo

---

[1] These scenarios are illustrative examples describing typical patients. They are not based on individual patients, but reflect current medical practice.

testing to assess their individual breast cancer predisposition (Siemens Healthcare Diagnostics Inc. 2008).

In contrast, Patient 2 has been diagnosed at age 40 with type 2 diabetes, an imprecise category that serves primarily to distinguish his disease from diabetes that typically occurs at younger ages (type 1) or during pregnancy (gestational). The diagnosis gives little insight into the specific molecular pathophysiology of the disease and its complications; similarly there is little basis for tailoring treatment to a patient's pathophysiology. The patient's internist will likely prescribe metformin, a drug used for over 50 years and still the most common treatment for type II diabetes in the United States. No concrete molecular information is available to customize Patient 2's therapy to reduce his risk for kidney failure, blindness or other diabetes-related complications. No tests are available to measure risk of diabetes for his siblings and children. Patient 2 and his family are not yet benefitting from today's explosion of information on the pathophysiology of disease (A.D.A.M. Medical Encyclopedia 2011; Gordon 2011; Kellett 2011).

What elements of our research and medical enterprise contribute to making the Patient 1 scenario exceptional, and Patient 2 typical? Could it be that something as fundamental as our current system for classifying diseases is actually *inhibiting* progress? Today's classification system is based largely on measurable "signs and symptoms," such as a breast mass or elevated blood sugar, together with descriptions of tissues or cells, and often fail to specify molecular pathways that drive disease or represent targets of treatment.[2] Consider a world where a diagnosis itself routinely provides insight into a specific pathogenic pathway. Consider a world where clinical information, including molecular features, becomes part of a vast "Knowledge Network of Disease" that would support precise diagnosis and individualized treatment. What if the potential of molecular features shared by seemingly disparate diseases to suggest radically new treatment regimens were fully realized? In such a world, a new, more accurate and precise "taxonomy of disease" could enable each patient to benefit from and contribute to what is known.

THE CHARGE TO THE COMMITTEE

In consideration of such possibilities, and at the request of the Director of the National Institutes of Health, an ad hoc Committee of the National Research Council was convened to explore the feasibility and need, and to develop a potential framework, for creating "a New Taxonomy of human diseases based on molecular biology" (Box 1-1). The Committee hosted a two- day workshop

---

[2] To clarify, the committee is not suggesting that all diseases would have an equally precise taxonomy, rather each disease should be classified, and treatment provided, using the best available molecular information about the mechanism of disease.

Box 1-1
Statement of Task

At the request of the Director's Office of NIH, an ad hoc Committee of the National Research Council will explore the feasibility and need, and develop a potential framework, for creating a "New Taxonomy" of human diseases based on molecular biology. As part of its deliberations, the Committee will host a large two-day workshop that convenes diverse experts in both basic and clinical disease biology to address the feasibility, need, scope, impact, and consequences of defining this New Taxonomy. The workshop participants will also consider the essential elements of the framework by addressing topics that include, but are not limited to:

• Compiling the huge diversity of extant data from molecular studies of human disease to assess what is known, identify gaps, and recommend priorities to fill these gaps.
• Developing effective and acceptable mechanisms and policies for selection, collection, storage, and management of data, as well as means to provide access to and interpret these data.
• Defining the roles and interfaces among the stakeholder communities— public and private funders, data contributors, clinicians, patients, industry, and others.
• Considering how to address the many ethical concerns that are likely to arise in the wake of such a program.

The Committee will also consider recommending a small number of case studies that might be used as an initial test for the framework.
The ad hoc Committee will use the workshop results in its deliberations as it develops recommendations for a framework in a consensus report. The report may form a basis for government and other research funding organizations regarding molecular studies of human disease. The report will not, however, include recommendations related to funding, government organization, or policy issues.

(see Appendix C) that convened diverse experts in both basic biology and clinical medicine to address the feasibility, need, scope, impact, and consequences of creating a "New Taxonomy of human diseases based on molecular biology". The information and opinions conveyed at the workshop informed and influenced an intensive series of Committee deliberations (in person and by teleconference) over a six-month period. The Committee emphasized that molecular biology was one important *base* of information for the "New Taxonomy", but not a limitation or constraint. Moreover, the Committee did not view its charge as prescribing a specific new disease nomenclature. Rather, the Committee saw its challenge as crafting a framework for integrating the rapidly expanding range and detail of biological, behavioral, and experiential information to facilitate basic discovery, and to drive the development of a more accurate and precise classification of disease (i.e., a "New Taxonomy"), which in turn will enable better medicine.

The vision for a New Taxonomy informed by the proposed "Knowledge Network" shares some similarities with the widely discussed concept of "Personalized Medicine," recently defined by the President's Council on Advisors on Science and Technology (PCAST) as "the tailoring of medical treatment to the individual characteristics of each patient . . . to classify individuals into subpopulations that differ in their susceptibility to a particular disease or their response to a specific treatment. Preventative or therapeutic interventions can then be concentrated on those who will benefit, sparing expense and side effects for those who will not" (PCAST 2008, p. 1). Others have used the related term "Precision Medicine" to refer to a very similar concept (see Glossary). Those who favor the latter term do so in part because it is less likely to be misinterpreted as meaning that each patient will be treated differently from every other patient. However, to be clear, the use of either term in this report refers to the PCAST definition.

A BRIEF HISTORY OF DISEASE TAXONOMIES

One of the first attempts to establish a scientific classification of disease was undertaken by Carolus Linnaeus, who developed the taxonomic system that is still used to classify living organisms. His 1763 publication *Genera Morborum* (Linné 1763) classified diseases into such categories as exanthematic (feverish with skin eruptions), phlogistic (feverish with heavy pulse and topical pain), and dolorous (painful). The effort was largely a failure because of the lack of an adequate understanding of the biological basis of disease. For example, without a germ theory of disease, rabies was characterized as a psychiatric disorder because of the brain dysfunction that occurs in advanced cases. This illustrates how a classification system for disease that is divorced from the biological basis of disease can mislead and impede efforts to develop better treatments.

Even 100 years ago, the *Manual of the International List of Causes of Death*, second revision, (Wilbur 1911), which over time would become the International Statistical Classification of Diseases and Related Health Problems (ICD), lumped lung cancer and brain cancer into the category of "cancer of other organs or not specified." No distinction was made between type 1 and type 2 diabetes, endocrine diseases were categorized under General Diseases, and categories existed for "nervous fever," "inanition," and "found dead."

Today, the ICD, which is currently in its tenth revision, remains the most commonly used categorization of disease (WHO 2007). Published by the World Health Organization (WHO), ICD-10 is used for statistical analyses, reimbursement, and decision support, making it an integral part of health-care systems throughout the world. As will be discussed, the ICD is currently undergoing a major revision, which will result in the publication of ICD-11 in approximately 2015.

THE TAXONOMIC NEEDS OF THE BIOMEDICAL
RESEARCH AND MEDICAL PRACTICE COMMUNITIES

Taxonomies underpin many health-related systems, such as the organization of the curriculum of medical education, the published biomedical literature,[3] textbooks, and disease coding systems such as the ICD. Although grounded in a scientific understanding of disease, taxonomies such as the ICD must address the needs of the ever-expanding public health and health-care delivery communities across the globe. Organizations such as WHO must have access to accurate and timely measures of disease incidence and prevalence in multiple continents to make recommendations. Similarly, the health-care industry in the United States depends on an accurate disease classification system to track the delivery of medical care and to determine reimbursement rates. Both of these communities rely on highly robust data collection practices to make decisions that can impact millions of individuals. In this context, a formalized nomenclature is essential for clear communication and understanding. The current practice of updating the ICD nomenclature periodically attempts to balance: (1) the need for a consistent terminology to permit clear communication about diseases that are defined by agreed upon criteria, with (2) the need to ensure that the classification system (i.e., the taxonomy) properly reflects advances in our understanding of molecular pathways and environmental factors that contribute to disease origin and pathology.

However, in part because it must serve the administrative needs of the public health and health-care delivery communities, the current ICD taxonomy is disconnected from much of the biomedical research community (see Figure 1-1). Indeed, few basic researchers know of the existence of ICD, and even fewer use this classification in any way. Thus, two extensive stakeholder groups, represented on one hand by biomedical researchers, and biotechnology and pharmaceutical industries, and on the other by clinicians, health agencies and payers, are widely perceived to be largely unrelated, and to have distinct interests and goals, and therefore taxonomic needs. This is unfortunate because new insights into human disease emerging from basic research and the explosion of information both in basic biology and medicine have the potential to revolutionize disease taxonomy, diagnosis, therapeutic development, and clinical decisions. However, more integration of the informational resources available to these diverse communities will be required before this potential can be fully realized

---

[3] For example, an information resource used extensively by both clinicians and researchers, PubMed/MEDLINE, is built on the MeSH terminology hierarchy of diseases.

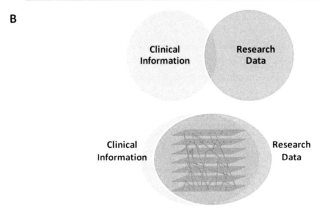

FIGURE 1-1 Integration would benefit all stakeholder communities.
(A) Different stakeholder communities are perceived to have distinct taxonomic and informational needs. (B) Integration of information and a consolidation of needs could better serve all stakeholders.
SOURCE: Committee on A Framework for Developing a New Taxonomy of Disease.

with the attendant benefits of more individualized treatments and improved outcomes for patients.

MISSED OPPORTUNITIES OF CURRENT TAXONOMIES

Currently used disease classifications have properties that limit their information content and usability. Most importantly, current disease taxonomies, including ICD-10, are primarily based on symptoms, on microscopic examination of diseased tissues and cells, and on other forms of laboratory and imaging studies and are not designed optimally to incorporate or exploit rapidly emerging molecular data, incidental patient characteristics, or socio-environmental influences on disease. The ability of current taxonomic systems to incorporate

---

Box 1-2
A Flexnerian Moment?

In 1910 educator Abraham Flexner released a report that revolutionized American medical education by advocating a commitment to professionalization, high academic standards, and close integration with basic science (Flexner 1910). The subsequent rise of academic medical centers with a strong emphasis on research—coupled, after World War II, with greatly expanded merit-based funding of research through the National Institutes of Health and other public and private entities—allowed the United States to capture global leadership in medical research, launch the biotechnology industry, and pioneer countless science-based innovations in health care.

The vast expansion of molecular knowledge currently underway could have benefits comparable to those that accompanied the professionalization of medicine and biomedical research in the early part of the 20th century. Indeed, during his talk at the Committee's workshop, Dr. Christopher G. Chute, a Mayo Clinic professor and leader in the development of ICD-11, said that the potential of the genomic transformation of medicine "far exceeds the introduction of antibiotics and aseptic surgery." However, achieving the full potential of the molecular revolution will require—and to an important extent enable—re-thinking both biomedical research and health care on a Flexnerian scale. Creation of a Knowledge Network of Disease that consolidates and integrates basic, clinical, social, and behavioral information, and that helps to inform a New Taxonomy that enables the delivery of improved, more individualized health care, will be a crucial element of this revolutionary change (Chute 2011).

---

fundamental knowledge is also limited by their basic structure. Taxonomies historically have relied on a hierarchical structure in which individual diseases are successively subdivided into types and subtypes. This rigid organizational structure precludes description of the complex interrelationships that link diseases to each other, and to the vast array of causative factors. It also can lead to the artificial separation of diseases based on distinct symptoms that have related underlying molecular mechanisms. For example, mutations in the *LMNA* gene give rise to a remarkably diverse set of diseases, including Emery-Dreyfus muscular dystrophy, Charcot-Marie-Tooth axonal neuropathy, lipodystrophy, and premature aging disorders. However, despite their remarkable genetic, molecular, and cellular similarities, these diseases are currently classified as distantly related. While this approach may have been adequate in an era when treatments were largely directed toward symptoms rather than underlying causes, there is a clear risk that continued reliance on hierarchical taxonomies will inhibit efforts—already successful in the case of some diseases—to exploit rapidly expanding mechanistic insights therapeutically.

A further limitation of taxonomic systems is the intrinsically static nature of their information content. The ICD system is designed to be updated every ten years with minor updates every three years. But many organizations are still working with ICD-9, which was released in 1977, even though ICD-10 was released in 1992. Because of the time it takes to implement ICD revisions in administrative systems, the current taxonomic system is perpetually outdated. Moreover, the static structure of current taxonomies does not lend itself to the continuous integration of new disease parameters as they become available. This is particularly troublesome given that new data regarding the molecular nature of disease are becoming available at an ever-increasing rate.

Current efforts to revise the ICD classification attempt to address these limitations. ICD-11 will be based on a foundational layer from which "linearizations" will be derived (Tu et al. 2010). While the linearizations will be relatively static and hierarchical, the foundational layer is being designed to support multi-parent hierarchies and connections, and to be updated continuously.[4] Importantly, the new classification will combine phenomenological characterization of phenotype with genomic factors that might explain or at least distinguish phenotypes.[5] Different lung cancers, for example, could be explicitly differentiated by genomic characterization. This is important because knowledge about the specific molecular pathways contributing to the biology of particular types of lung cancer can be used to guide selection of the most appropriate treatment for such patients.

Although the release of ICD-11 will mark an important step forward, the Committee thinks that the amount of information available for this effort can be vastly increased by a two-stage process leading to a Knowledge Network of Disease. As discussed in detail in following sections of this report, the first stage in developing this Knowledge Network would involve creating an Information Commons containing a combination of molecular data, medical histories (including information about social and physical environments), and health outcomes for large numbers of individual patients. The Committee envisions this stage occurring in conjunction with the ongoing delivery of clinical care to these patients, rather than in specialized settings specifically crafted for research purposes. The second stage, the construction of the Knowledge Network itself,

---

[4] The ICD-11 revision process is closely coordinated with SNOMED—the Systematized Nomenclature of Medicine developed by the International Health Terminology Standards Development Organization (IHTSDO). SNOMED is a large, clinically focused ontology that uses high-level nodes to aggregate more granular data. The WHO and IHTSDO have signed a memorandum of understanding so that the two systems will be complementary rather than competing. The intent is to harmonize the two systems so that the aggregation layer of SNOMED corresponds to ICD-11 and the extensions of ICD-11 become elements of SNOMED.

[5] It should be noted that the International Classification of Diseases for Oncology (ICD-O) already attempts to capture genomic data relevant to disease definitions. The third series of the WHO Monographs on the Pathology and Genetics of Tumours sought to integrate genomic data, where available, into disease definitions and indeed today many tumor types are molecularly defined (Vardiman et al. 2009;. Campo et al. 2011; Travis et al. 2011).

would involve data mining of the Information Commons and integration of these data with the scientific literature—specifically with evolving knowledge of the fundamental biological mechanisms underlying disease.

Such a Knowledge Network of Disease would enable development of a more molecularly-based taxonomy. This "New Taxonomy" could, for example, lead to more specific diagnosis and targeted therapies for muscular dystrophy patients based on the specific mutations in their genes. In other cases, it could suggest targeted therapies for patients with the same genetic mechanism of disease despite very different clinical presentations.

AN INFORMATION COMMONS, A KNOWLEDGE NETWORK, AND A NEW TAXONOMY THAT WOULD INTEGRATE MANY TYPES OF INFORMATION AND SERVE ALL STAKEHOLDERS

As will be described later in the report, the Committee envisions that the Information Commons, which would underlie the Knowledge Network of Disease and the New Taxonomy, would have some analogies with geographical information systems (GISs), which are designed to capture, store, manipulate, and analyze all types of geographically referenced data and make them widely accessible in applications (ESRI 1990) such as Google Maps (Figure 1-2). Most

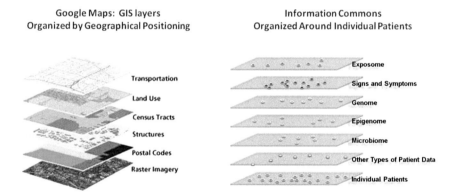

FIGURE 1-2 An Information Commons might use a GIS-type structure.
The proposed, individual-centric Information Commons (right panel) is somewhat analogous to a layered GIS (left panel). In both cases, the bottom layer defines the organization of all the overlays. However, in a GIS, any vertical line through the layers connects related snippets of information since all the layers are organized by geographical position. In contrast, data in each of the higher layers of the Information Commons will overlay on the patient layer in complex ways (e.g., patients with similar microbiomes and symptoms may have very different genome sequences).
SOURCE: FPA 2011 (left panel).

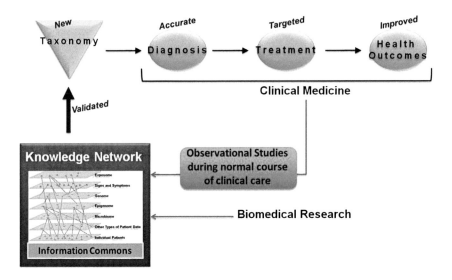

FIGURE 1-3 A knowledge network of disease would enable a new taxonomy.
An individual-centric Information Commons, in combination with all extant biological knowledge, will inform a Knowledge Network of Disease, which will capture the
exceedingly complex causal influences and pathogenic mechanisms that determine
an individual's health. The Knowledge Network of Disease would allow researchers
to hypothesize new intralayer cluster and interlayer connections. Validated findings
that emerge from the Knowledge Network, such as those which define new diseases or
subtypes of diseases that are clinically relevant (e.g., which have implications for patient
prognosis or therapy) would be incorporated into the New Taxonomy to improve diagnosis and treatment.
SOURCE: Committee on A Framework for Developing a New Taxonomy of Disease.

users would interact with these resources at the higher-value-added levels,
the Knowledge Network and the New Taxonomy, rather than at the level of
the underlying Information Commons (Figure 1-3). Investigators using the
Knowledge Network of Disease could propose hypotheses about the importance of various inter- and intra-layer connections that contribute to disease
origin, severity, or progression, or that support the subclassification of particular diseases into those with different molecular mechanisms, prognoses, and/
or treatments, and these ideas then could be tested in an attempt to establish
their validity, reproducibility, and robustness. Validated findings that emerge
from the Knowledge Network of Disease and are shown to be useful for defining new diseases or subtypes of diseases that are clinically relevant (e.g., which
have implications for patient prognosis or therapy) could be incorporated into
the New Taxonomy to improve diagnosis and treatment. Whether the "New

Taxonomy" that is informed and refined by the Knowledge Network of Disease would best be realized as a modification of the ICD taxonomy, or should represent an entirely distinct taxonomy that exists in parallel with ICD and other taxonomies, will depend on a number of factors. However, in either case, the goal of basing the New Taxonomy on the Knowledge Network of Disease will be to improve markedly the quantity and quality of information that can be used in biomedicine for the basic discovery of disease mechanisms, improved disease classification, and better medical care.

RATIONALE AND ORGANIZATION OF THE REPORT

Today, historic forces are transforming biomedical research and health care. Information technology, clinical medicine, and the public attitudes that govern the ways that science, medicine, and society interact are all in flux.

A Knowledge Network of Disease could embrace and inform rapidly expanding efforts by the biomedical research community to define at the molecular level the disease predispositions and pathogenic processes occurring in individuals. This network has the potential to play a critical role across the globe for the public-health and health-care-delivery communities by enabling development of a more accurate, molecularly-informed taxonomy of disease.

This report lays out the case for developing such a Knowledge Network of Disease and associated New Taxonomy. Chapter 2 asks "Why now?" It examines basic trends in research, information technology, clinical medicine, and public attitudes that have created an unprecedented opportunity to influence biomedical research and health-care delivery in ways that will benefit all stakeholders.

Chapter 3 asks "What would a Knowledge Network of Disease and New Taxonomy look like?" It describes why the system needs to be dynamic, continuously evolving, integrative, and flexible, and why it needs to enable interrogation by a wide range of users, from basic scientists to clinicians, health-care workers, and the general public.

Chapter 4 asks "How do we get there?" It describes the need for a series of pilot studies to evaluate the feasibility of creating an individual-centric Information Commons and deriving a Knowledge Network and New Taxonomy from it, and to begin to explore the utility of these resources for improving individual health outcomes. This chapter also addresses the impediments that need to be overcome and changes in medical education that will be required before the Knowledge Network of Disease and resulting New Taxonomy can be expected to achieve their full potential for improving human health.

In Chapter 5, the report closes with an epilogue that summarizes the Committee's rationale for its recommendations and describes how the new resources described in this report could serve the needs of basic scientists, translational researchers, policy makers, insurers, medical trainees, clinicians, and patients.

2

Why Now?

The rise of data-intensive biology, advances in information technology, and changes in the way health care is delivered have created a compelling opportunity to improve the diagnosis and treatment of disease by developing a Knowledge Network, and associated New Taxonomy, that would integrate biological, patient, and outcomes data on a scale hitherto beyond our reach. Key enablers of this opportunity include:

- New capabilities to compile molecular data on patients on a scale that was unimaginable 20 years ago.
- Increasing success in utilizing molecular information to improve the diagnosis and treatment of disease.
- Advances in information technology, such as the advent of electronic health records, that make it possible to acquire detailed clinical information about large numbers of individual patients and to search for unexpected correlations within enormous datasets.
- A "perfect storm" among stakeholders that has increased receptivity to fundamental changes throughout the biomedical research and health-care-delivery systems.
- Shifting public attitudes toward molecular data and privacy of health-care information.

Scientific research, information technology, medicine, and public attitudes are all undergoing unprecedented changes. Biology has acquired the capacity to systematically compile molecular data on a scale that was unimaginable 20 years ago. Diverse technological advances make it possible to gather, integrate, analyze, and disseminate health-related biological data in ways that could greatly advance both biomedical research and clinical care. Meanwhile, the magnitude of the challenges posed by the sheer scientific complexity of the molecular influences on health and disease are becoming apparent and suggest the need for powerful new research resources. All these changes provide an opportunity for the biomedical science and clinical communities to come together to improve both the discovery of new knowledge and health-care delivery. As discussed in this chapter, the Committee concluded that this opportunity could best be exploited through a major, long-term commitment to create an Information Commons, a Knowledge Network of Disease, and a New Taxonomy.

BIOLOGY HAS BECOME A DATA-INTENSIVE SCIENCE

Advances in DNA-sequencing technology powerfully illustrate biology's conversion to a data-intensive science. The first papers describing practical methods of DNA sequencing were published in 1977 (Maxam and Gilbert 1977; Sanger et al. 1977). These methods required radioisotopic labeling of DNA, hand-crafting of large electrophoretic gels, and considerable expertise with biochemical and recombinant-DNA techniques. Although the impact of these early DNA-sequencing methods on biological discovery was profound, the total amount of sequence deposited in GenBank, the central depository for such data, did not pass one billion base pairs (one-third of the length of a single human genome) until 1997 (NCBI 2011a), and it only reached this landmark after a first generation of automated instruments came into widespread use (Favello et al. 1995). Since then > 300 billion base pairs (Benson et al. 2011) have been deposited, illustrating the still ongoing explosion of genomic data in the last 20 years.

The National Human Genome Research Institute estimated that the total cost of obtaining a single human-genome sequence in 2001 was $95 million (Wetterstrand 2011; see Figure 2-1). Costs subsequently dropped exponentially following a trajectory described in electronics as Moore's Law, connoting a reduction of cost by 50 percent every two years, until the spring of 2007, at which point the estimated cost of a single human-genome sequence was still nearly $10 million. At that point, introduction of a second generation of automated DNA-sequencing instruments, based on massively parallel, miniaturized analysis, led to a collapse in costs far faster than the Moore's Law projection. The most recent update, in January 2011, estimates the cost of a complete-genome sequence at $21,000, and the cost is still dropping rapidly, with a "$1000 genome" becoming a realistic target within a few years. (Wolinsky 2007; MITRE Corporation 2010; Mardis 2011)While whole-genome sequencing remains expensive by the standards of most clinical laboratory tests, the trend-line leaves little doubt that costs will drop into the range of many routine clinical tests within a few years. Whole-genome sequencing will soon become cheaper than many of the specific genetic tests that are widely ordered today and ultimately

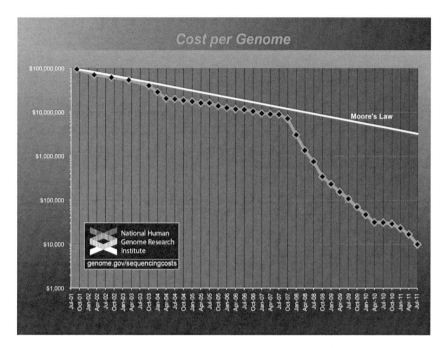

FIGURE 2-1 The plummeting cost of complete genome sequencing.
The cost of complete genome sequencing is falling faster than Moore's Law. The cost is still dropping rapidly, with a "$1000 genome" becoming a realistic target within a few years.
SOURCE: Wetterstrand 2011.

will likely become trivial compared to the cost of routine medical care. Hence, the costs of DNA sequencing will soon cease to be a limiting factor (MITRE Corporation 2010). Instead, the clinical utility of genome sequences and public acceptance of their use will drive future developments.

Admittedly, the cost trajectory of DNA sequencing is an unusual success story, even by high-tech standards. However, it is by no means unique: parallel developments in other areas of molecular analysis, such as the analysis of large numbers of small-molecule metabolites and proteins, and the detection of single molecules, are likely to sweep away purely economic barriers to the diffusion of many data-intensive molecular methods into biomedical research and clinical medicine. These technologies will make it possible to monitor and ultimately to understand and predict the functioning of complex molecular networks in health and disease.

THE OPPORTUNITY TO INTEGRATE
DATA-INTENSIVE BIOLOGY WITH MEDICINE

Human physiology is far more complex than any known machine. The molecular idiosyncrasies of each human being underlie both the exhilarating potential and daunting challenges associated with "personalized medicine". Individual humans typically differ from each other at millions of sites in their genomes (Ng et al. 2009). More than ten thousand of these differences are known to have the potential to alter physiology, and this estimate is certain to grow as our understanding of the genome expands. All of this new genetic information could potentially improve diagnosis and treatment of diseases by taking into account individual differences among patients. We now have the technology to identify these genetic differences—and, in some instances, infer their consequences for disease risk and treatment response. Some successes along these lines have already occurred; however, the scale of these efforts is currently limited by the lack of the infrastructure that would be required to integrate molecular information with electronic medical records during the ordinary course of health care.

The human microbiome project represents an additional opportunity to inform human health care. The microorganisms that live inside and on humans are estimated to outnumber human somatic cells by a factor of ten. "If humans are thought of as a composite of microbial and human cells", then "the human genetic landscape is an aggregate of the genes in the human genome and the microbiome, and human metabolic features" are "a blend of human and microbial traits" (Turnbaugh et al. 2007). A growing list of diseases, including obesity, inflammatory bowel disease, gastrointestinal cancers, eczema, and psoriasis, have been associated with changes in the structure or function of human microbiota. The ultimate goal of studying the human microbiome is to better understand the impact of microbial variation across individuals and populations and to use this information to target the human microbiome with antibiotics, probiotics, and prebiotics as therapies for specific disorders. While this field is in its infancy, growing knowledge of the human microbiome and its function will enable disease classification and medicine to encompass both humans and their resident microbes.

There are already compelling examples of improvements in patient care that have emerged from studies of the human genome and human microbiome:

- Some patients with high cholesterol are heterozygous for a non-functional variant of the low-density-lipoprotein-receptor gene, a genotype found in one out of every 500 individuals. Lifestyle interventions alone are ineffective in these individuals at reducing the likelihood of early-onset cardiovascular disease (Huijgen et al. 2008). Consequently, the ability to identify the patients who carry the non-functional receptor makes it possible to proceed directly to the use of statin drugs at an early age, rather than first attempting to control cholesterol with diet and exercise. There is strong evidence that the early use of statin drugs in these individuals can provide a therapeutic benefit.

- In the United States it is estimated that 0.06 percent of the population carries mutations in the tumor suppressor *BRCA1* and 0.4 percent of people carry mutations in *BRCA2* (Malone et al. 2006). These mutations predispose to cancer, particularly breast and ovarian cancer (King et al. 2003). Women who carry these mutations can reduce their risk of death from cancer through increased cancer screening or through prophylactic surgeries to remove their breasts or ovaries (Roukos and Briasoulis 2007); until these mutations were identified it was not possible to determine who carried the mutations or to take proactive steps to manage risk.

- Lung cancer patients can now be separated by the genetic profiles of their cancers into distinct groups that benefit from different treatments (see Box 2-1).

- It is now clear that most cases of stomach ulcers, once thought to be caused by stress and other non-infectious factors, are due to colonization of the stomach lining with the *Helicobacter pylori* bacterium, which is very common in human populations (Atherton 2006). This finding has radically changed the treatment of this disorder. *H. pylori* infection also is thought to predispose to the development of stomach cancer, suggesting that treatment of this infection can both help cure gastric ulcers and also may reduce the development of cancer of the stomach. In addition, epidemiological studies and other data have raised the possibility that *H. pylori* infection may reduce the individual's likelihood of developing allergic diseases or even obesity (Blaser and Falkow 2009), suggesting that the full complexity of the relationship between infection with this organism and human health and disease remains to be determined.

- In the last decade, genetic analyses have allowed a more precise diagnostic classification of type 2 diabetes. Children and young adults with mild glucose intolerance and often a strong family history of diabetes were previously categorized as having "Maturity Onset Diabetes of the Young (MODY)". MODY is now understood to represent a series of specific genetic variants that affect pancreatic beta cell function (Fajans et al. 2001) such that the American Diabetes Association classification of type 2 diabetes has replaced the descriptive term MODY with the specific genetic defects (e.g., chromosome 7, glucokinase; chromosome 12, hepatic nuclear factor 1—alpha; etc.) A dynamic, continuously evolving Knowledge Network of Disease will be needed to accommodate future additions to this list of specific genetic predispositions to

Box 2-1
Distinguishing Types of Lung Cancer

Lung cancer is the leading cause of cancer-related death in the United States as well as worldwide, causing more than one million total deaths annually (ACS 2011). Traditionally, lung cancers have been divided into two main types based on the tumors' histological appearance: small-cell lung cancer and non-small-cell lung cancer. Non-small-cell lung cancer is comprised of three subgroups, each of them defined by histology, including adenocarcinoma, squamous-cell carcinoma, and large-cell carcinoma.

Since 2004, knowledge of the molecular drivers of non-small-cell lung cancer has exploded (Figure 2-2). Drivers are mutations in genes that contribute to inappropriate cellular proliferation. These driver mutations are necessary for tumor formation and tumor maintenance. If the inappropriate function of the mutant protein is shut down, dramatic anti-tumor effects can ensue.

In 2004 two drugs were in development, Gefitinib and Erlotinib, which inhibited the function of certain receptor tyrosine kinases, including epidermal growth factor receptor (EGFR). These receptors were known to send signals that promote cellular proliferation and survival, and increased signaling was thought to contribute to some cancers. In early trials, the drugs were shown to produce dramatic anti-tumor effects in about 10 percent of patients with non-small-cell lung cancer (MSKCC 2005). Other patients did not appear to respond at all. However, the dramatic tumor shrinkage in some patients was enough for U.S. Food and Drug Administration approval in 2003, even though the molecular basis for the response was then unknown. Without the ability to recognize the responding patients as a biologically distinct subset, these agents were tried unsuccessfully on a broad range of lung-cancer patients, doing nothing for most patients other than increasing costs and side effects. In retrospect, some clinical trials with these agents probably failed because the actual responders represented too small a proportion of the patients in the trials (Pao and Miller 2005).

Subsequently, it was discovered that the responding patients carried mutations that activated EGFR in their cancers (Kris et al. 2003; Lynch et al. 2004; Paez et al. 2004; Pao et al. 2004). This made it possible to predict which patients would respond to the therapy and to administer the therapy only to this subset of patients. This led to the design of much more effective clinical trials as well as reduced treatment costs and increased treatment effectiveness.

Since then, many studies have further divided lung cancers into subsets that can be defined by driver mutations. Not all of these driver mutations can currently be targeted with drugs and cancer cells are quick to develop resistance to targeted drugs even when they are available. Nonetheless, this recent information makes it possible to develop new targeted therapies that can extend and improve the quality of life for cancer patients.

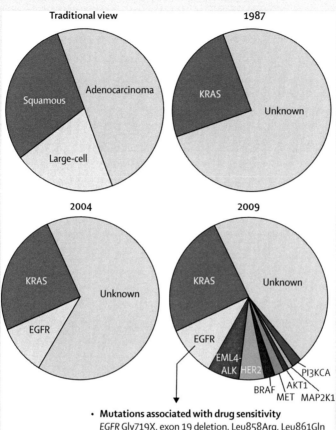

FIGURE 2-2 Knowledge of non-small-cell lung cancer has evolved substantially in recent decades.

The traditional characterization of lung cancers based on histology has been replaced over the past 20 years by classifications based on driver mutations. In 1987, this classification was rudimentary as only one driver mutation had been identified, KRAS. However, the sophistication of this system for molecular classification has improved with the advent of more genetic information and the identification of many more driver mutations. Similar approaches could improve the diagnosis, classification, and treatment of many other diseases.

SOURCE: Pao and Girard 2011.

in type 2 diabetes (with the vision of adding clarity to the diagnosis of Patient 2).

The human genome and microbiome projects are only two examples of emerging biological information that has the potential to inform health care. It is similarly likely that other molecular data (such as epigenetic or metabolomic data), information on the patient's history of exposure to environmental agents, and psychosocial or behavioral information will all need to be incorporated into a Knowledge Network and New Taxonomy that would enhance the diagnosis and treatment of disease.

THE URGENT NEED TO BETTER UNDERSTAND PHENOTYPE-GENOTYPE CORRELATIONS

While dramatic progress in understanding the relationship between molecular features and phenotype is being made, there is an urgent need to understand these links better and to develop strategies to deal with their implications for the individual patient. *BRCA1* and *BRCA2* genes are a good example. The discovery of mutations in *BRCA1* and *BRCA2* in some people made it possible to identify individuals at increased risk of cancer, allowing them to manage their risk with increased cancer screening and prophylactic surgeries. A database cataloging *BRCA1* mutations recently listed 2,136 distinct variants of the gene (NHGRI 2011). Of these, 1,167 were judged by the database's curators as likely to be clinically significant, while most of the rest were categorized as of "unknown" clinical significance. Among the mutations that are believed to be clinically significant, some are thought to confer a higher risk of cancer than others (Gayther et al. 1995) but there remains uncertainty about the extent to which most mutations increase cancer risk (Fackenthal and Olopade 2007).

As a consequence, people with *BRCA1* and *BRCA2* mutations are forced to make life-altering treatment decisions with incomplete information. To what extent does their mutation increase their risks of breast and ovarian cancer and how do these risks change with age? Should they have prophylactic mastectomies or oophorectomies, and if so, when? Should they wait until after childbearing and how would that affect their risks? All of these real-life decisions carry heavy personal consequences as well as implications for health-care costs.

These treatment decisions do not need to be made based on such fragmentary information. If all patients who test positive for *BRCA1* or *BRCA2* mutations were tracked by their health-care providers long term, it would be possible to determine what percentage of patients with each mutation develop cancer, and which cancers. It would be possible to assess the extent to which prophylactic surgeries reduced risk. It would be possible to assess the effectiveness of increased cancer screening, the best ways to screen these patients, and the complications that arise from the inevitable false-positive results that come from increased screening. Efforts along these lines have so far been based on modest numbers of patients or cohorts that are not fully representative of the larger population because it has not been practical to integrate genetic information, treatment decisions, and outcomes data for large numbers of unselected patients. However, recent advances in genomic and information technologies now make it possible to address systematically these issues by integrating large datasets that already exist (see Box 2-2).

BRCA1 and *BRCA2* are only two of many genes in which differences between individuals have significant implications for disease risk and treatment decisions. We have approximately 20,000 genes in our genome and many of these genes may have many disease-relevant alleles, just like *BRCA1*. Even if only a subset of this variation has significant implications for disease risk or treatment response we have the potential to improve the detection, diagnosis, and treatment of disease dramatically by large-scale efforts to assess phenotype-genotype correlations. By integrating patient genotype with health information and outcomes data a New Taxonomy could identify many new genetic variants with significant implications for health care.

There is every reason to expect that the genetic influences on most common diseases will be complex. In each patient, variants in multiple genes will affect disease onset, progression, and response to treatment, and long-term environmental modulation of these processes will be the rule rather than the exception. While recent breakthroughs have focused on genomics as a consequence of the rapid development of technology in that area, the future may see comparable advances in our ability to understand epigenetic, environmental, microbial, and social contributions to disease risk and progression. Under these circumstances, there is an obvious need to categorize diseases with finer granularity, greater reference to the underlying biology, and in the context of a dynamic Knowledge Network that has the capacity to integrate the new information on many levels. Unraveling these diverse influences on human diseases will be a major scientific challenge of the 21st century.

DRAMATIC ADVANCES IN INFORMATION TECHNOLOGY ARE DRIVING SYSTEMIC CHANGE

The United States and other countries are currently making multibillion-dollar investments to implement electronic health records (EHRs) to improve clinical care. The development of such records creates several new opportunities to integrate health-care information and biological data and to search for new links between clinical test results, patient data, and outcomes.

- The increased functionality of EHRs and the improved performance of search tools open the door to conduct large cohort studies on a wide range of diseases. Patients with characteristics of interest—for

Box 2-2
Prospective Cohort Studies—A Special Role

Much of our knowledge about "risk factors" that predispose to complex diseases comes from observational epidemiological studies, either case-control studies in which aspects of the life experience of a series of cases are compared with those of appropriate controls, or prospective cohort studies in which large numbers of people are followed over time and the life experience of those who develop a specific disease are compared with those of the much larger number who have not.

For example, much of what is known about the predictive value of biochemical factors that are measured in plasma or serum, such as the relation of cholesterol or other lipid with risk of heart attack, is derived from prospective cohort studies such as the Framingham Heart Study (FHS). Prospective studies are particularly valuable because the occurrence or treatment of disease may alter the levels of the biochemical factors so that inference based on levels measured in a series of already diagnosed cases may be biased. These biomarkers can be combined with information on lifestyle risk factors such as smoking and body mass index, and measurements that may also change after diagnosis such as blood pressure, to create a risk score such as the Framingham Risk Score, that is widely used to predict the 10-year risk of heart attack (Anderson et al. 1991). The Risk Score was based on data from slightly more than 5,500 subjects, among whom several hundred coronary heart disease (CHD) events occurred. A study of this size is adequate for relatively common disease events such as CHD, or quantitative traits such as blood pressure or bone density for which every participant has

example, those with rheumatoid arthritis or lacking response to antidepressants—could be selected via EHRs. Patients in these groups could then be recruited to provide samples or have their discarded clinical samples analyzed for research.

- EHRs could be used to provide additional clinical characterization or to help fill in missing details on subjects studied in a cohort or biobank. In either case, the result would be a rich clinical characterization of patients at low cost and with linkages to corresponding biological samples that can be used for molecular studies. Research questions could be addressed faster and at lower cost as compared to the current standard practice of designing large, labor-intensive prospective studies.

- EHRs permit longitudinal analyses of data from millions of people. When linked with genomic information—yielding what has been called EHR genomic research—EHRs could provide the large numa value, but too small to provide enough cases of less common diseases such as site-specific cancers. Larger prospective cohort studies such as the Nurses' Health Study (Missmer et al. 2004), and the European Prospective Investigation into Cancer (EPIC) (Kaaks et al. 2005), have explored the relationship between circulating steroid hormone levels and risk of breast cancer in cohorts of tens of thousands of women, with many hundreds of cases, but the number of cases occurring in the FHS is still relatively small due to the smaller size of the cohort. For risk factors with small effects, or to study the interactions between multiple risk factors, even the largest cohort studies may have too few cases to generate statistical power, and consortia such as the NCI Breast & Prostate Cohort Consortium (Campa et al. 2005) are needed to generate the thousands of cases necessary for adequate power. For less common diseases, consortia are again needed as no single study will have enough cases.

Some countries have established very large prospective cohort studies such as the UK Biobank (about 500,000 persons) (Palmer 2007), and some have advocated for a similar study in the United States (Collins 2004). However, the cost of enrolling half a million or more persons in a such a research study in the US, tracking them over decades, and obtaining information on medical diagnoses for a research database are estimated to be several billion dollars (Willett et al. 2007), even if the many feasibility issues can be overcome.

An Information Commons and Knowledge Network with appropriate informatic and consent mechanisms could generate similar large longitudinal sample sets and data through the provision of regular medical care, rather than considering these as research studies external to the health systems.

bers of subjects and detailed information needed to resolve many of the questions that smaller cohorts cannot address.

While the use of data from EHRs faces many difficulties, none of these difficulties is insurmountable. The cost advantages and potential to advance clinical care make expanding and accelerating studies using EHRs a high priority. Several health-care systems in the United States have started accruing large EHR databases linked to clinical biosamples. Notable among the U.S. efforts are the Harvard University/Partners Healthcare i2b2 effort, the Vanderbilt BioVu effort (Roden et al. 2008), the UCSF-Kaiser collaboration (discussed in Chapter 4) and the multi-center eMERGE Network (McCarty et al. 2011) (see Box 2-3).

Since EHR systems cover a broad swath of human illness, they provide a unique research opportunity to explore genotype-phenotype associations across many diseases. As articulated by Jones et al. (2005) and implemented by Denny et al. (2010), all diseases can be scanned using EHRs for significant associations with any genetic variant or set of variants. For example, a single genetic variant (e.g., a single nucleotide polymorphism or SNP) associated with diabetes in a standard genetics study can be promptly assessed for correlation with every EHR-derived phenotype such as obesity, heart disease, smoking history, and hypothyroidism. This approach has been colloquially termed PheWAS (Phenome-Wide Association Study), in contrast with the more widely developed approach

---

Box 2-3
The eMERGE Consortium

The Electronic Medical Records and Genomics (eMERGE) Network (www.gwas.org) is an NIH-funded consortium of five institutions with DNA data linked to electronic medical records. (All of the institutions agreed to contribute their genomic association results to dbGAP at the National Library of Medicine.) The goal of the consortium is to assess the utility of electronic medical records (EMRs) as resources for genomic science. The project includes an ethics component, community engagement, and the use of natural language processingto interpret EMRs. Each institution individually had proposed a genome-wide association study (GWAS) of about 3,000 subjects with a particular phenotype of interest (e.g. type 2 diabetes, cataracts, dementia, heart disease, and peripheral vascular disease) and an associated comparison group.

Several important lessons have been learned from the consortium's experience. First, patient data, obtained during the normal course of clinical care, has proven to be a valid source for replicating genome-phenome associations that previously had been reported only in carefully qualified research cohorts. Second, although the individual institutions initially thought that they had large enough effect sizes and odds ratios to be adequately powered, in most cases, the entire network was needed to determine genome-wide association. Third, high-quality EMR-derived phenotypes require four elements: codes (including ICD codes, though codes have to be repeated multiple times to gain validity), laboratory-medicine results, medication histories, and natural language processing of physician comments. The ability to extract high-quality phenotypes from narrative text is essential along with codes, laboratory results, and medication histories to get high predictive values. Fourth, although the five electronic medical systems have widely varying structures, coding systems, user interfaces, and users, once validated at one site, the information transported across the network with almost no degradation of its specificity and precision.

Another lesson of critical importance was that the major impediments that the eMERGE Consortium has had to address are policy related, rather than technical. For instance, a particular challenge has been to achieve both meaningful data sharing and respect for patient privacy concerns, while adhering to applicable regulations and laws (Kho et al. 2011; Masys 2011; McGuire et al. 2011) (eMERGE has addressed this issue, in part, by developing a simplified Data Use Agreement—see Appendix D.)

called GWAS (Genome-Wide Association Study). Such a scan may show that the original association is either an epiphenomenon of another pathology or part of a broader pathotype (Loscalzo et al. 2007). This approach provides an opportunity to explore this broader range of pathological mechanisms across a variety of disease types, which is not possible in single phenotype studies. The power of such association studies to detect relationships between genotype and disease is limited by the granularity and precision of the current taxonomic system for disease. A knowledge-network-derived taxonomy that distinguishes diseases with different biological drivers would enhance the power of association studies to uncover new insights.

GATHERING INFORMATION FROM INFORMAL DATA SOURCES

The explosive growth of social networks, particularly in the context of healthcare issues, may also serve as a novel source of data on health and disease. Evidence is already accumulating that these alternative and "informal" sources of health-care data, including information shared by individuals from ubiquitous technologies such as smart phones and social networks, can contribute significantly to collecting disease and health data (Brownstein et al. 2008, 2009, 2010a,b).

Many data sources exist outside of traditional health-care records that could be extremely useful in biomedical research and medical practice. Informal reports from large groups of people (also known as "crowd sourcing"), when properly filtered and refined, can produce data complementary to information from traditional sources. One example is the use of information from the web to detect the spread of disease in a population. In one instance, a system called HealthMap, which crawls about 50,000 websites each hour using a fully automated process, was able to detect an unusual respiratory illness in Veracruz, Mexico, weeks before traditional public-health agencies (Brownstein et al. 2009). It also was able to track the progression and spread of H1N1 on a global scale when no particular public-health agency or health-care resource could produce that kind of a picture.

The use of mobile phones also has tremendous potential, especially with developers building apps that engage patient populations. For example, a recent app called Outbreaks Near Me allows people to use their cell phones to learn about all the disease events in their neighborhood. People also can report back to the system, putting their own health information into the system.

Many of the social networking sites built around medical conditions are patient specific and allow individuals to share unstructured information about health outcomes. Mining that information within proper ethical guidelines provides a novel opportunity to monitor health outcomes. For example, Google has mined de-identified search data to build a picture of flu trends. The advent of these inexpensive ways of collecting health information creates new opportunities to integrate information that will enhance the diagnosis and treatment of disease.

INTEGRATING CLINICAL MEDICINE AND BASIC SCIENCE

Traditionally, a physician's office or clinic has had few direct connections with academic research laboratories. In this environment, patient-oriented research—particularly if it involved studying patients or patient-derived samples with state-of-the-art scientific techniques and experimental designs—required a major division of labor between the research and clinical settings. Typically, researchers have used informal referral networks to make contact with physicians caring for patients with diseases of special interest to the researchers. Once enrolled in a research study, the patient—or, in some cases, simply a tissue sample and a little clinical information—passed into a research setting that maintained its own infrastructure, including Institutional Review Boards (IRBs), patient coordinators, clinical evaluation centers, instrumentation, laboratory facilities, and data analysis centers. This approach often yielded descriptive and anecdotal results of uncertain relevance to larger (and more diverse) patient populations. Moreover, the patients who contributed are unlikely to remain connected to the research process or be aware of outcomes.[1] This research model is ill-suited to long-term follow-up of patients since it was never designed for this purpose.

Although remarkably successful in addressing its original goals of testing clearly defined hypotheses, this traditional approach to clinical research is poorly suited to answering current questions about human health that are often more open-ended and larger in scope than those typically addressed in the past. Based on committee experience and the input from multiple stakeholders during the course of this study, including the two-day workshop, the Committee identified several reasons that current study designs are mismatched to current needs. Traditional designs:

- **Require very large sample sizes—hence most studies are inevitably under-powered.** As emphasized above, the number and complexity of questions inherent in genotype-phenotype correlations is virtually unbounded. Patients with particularly informative genotypes and phenotypes—often difficult or impossible to recognize in advance—will typically be rare. Identification and recruitment of such patients in sufficient numbers to acquire clinically actionable information about their

---

[1] There are notable exceptions such as the Framingham Heart Study and Nurses' Health Study, which were designed from the outset to follow a cohort of patients over an extended period of time. See Box 2-2: Prospective Cohort Studies—A Special Role.

diseases will be possible only if molecular and clinical information can be combined in huge patient cohorts.

- **Involve high costs that are largely unnecessary because of increasing redundancy between the infrastructure present in research and clinical settings.** Most of what is needed to carry out data-intensive molecular studies of huge patient populations already exists in the health-care system or, increasingly, will exist as large coordinated health-care organizations absorb increasing portions of the patient population, EHRs are more widely implemented, medical decisions are increasingly driven by molecular analyses (particularly in the realm of oncology, but increasingly in other subspecialties as well), and consent standards for treatment converge with those for both outcomes and molecular research.

- **Encourage building closed rather than open research systems.** Researchers who devote their careers to building the research infrastructure described above, cultivating the physician networks, and navigating the IRB process have little incentive to share patient samples and data widely. Indeed, the suite of obstacles that a young investigator must overcome to penetrate this system are a major disincentive for involvement in patient-oriented research. In addition, the many talented biomedical researchers who choose to focus their work on model organisms (such as flies, worms, and mice) have little opportunity to share insights or collaborate with clinical researchers.

- **Leave most researchers and physicians living in separate, largely disconnected communities.** The current biomedical training system separates researchers and physicians from the earliest stages of their education and creates silos of specialized, but limited knowledge. The insular nature of the current biomedical system does not encourage interdisciplinary collaborations and has significant negative effects on training, study design, prioritization of research efforts, and translation of new research findings.

- **Are poorly suited to long-term follow-up of patients.** Long-term follow-up was not required to conduct the first generation of genotype-phenotype studies. The questions under investigation were typically of the nature "Do all cystic fibrosis patients have loss-of-function mutations in the *CFTR* gene?" Therefore, researchers who sought to establish the causal role of genotypes in particular phenotypes only needed confidence that patients had been correctly diagnosed. However, questions such as "Do cystic fibrosis patients with particular genotypes do better over a period of decades with particular treatments?" require long-term follow-up.

- **May not provide feedback on clinically relevant results for integration into a patient's clinical care.** To the extent that inherited germline variation and/or somatic genomic patterns are predictive of prognosis or response, the feedback of results to the clinical care of the individual research subjects may or may not occur according to a complex mixture of factors including the original informed-consent documents, the logistics of re-contacting subjects, the perceived validity of the scientific results (which may change over time), the time that has elapsed between when a sample was taken and the results were generated, and whether the laboratory work was performed under protocols that permit results feedback. These limiting factors mean that most research results are not integrated into clinical care. Expert opinion on the "duty to inform" research participants of clinically relevant results vary widely. Indeed, many researchers are reluctant to contribute data to a common resource as it may expose them to questions about whether feedback to participants is necessary or desirable.

For these, and many other reasons, the project of developing an Information Commons, a Knowledge Network of disease, and a New Taxonomy requires a long-term perspective. In a sense, this challenge has parallels with the building of Europe's great cathedrals–studies started by one generation will be completed by another, and plans will change over time as new techniques are developed and knowledge evolves. As costs in the health-care system are increasingly dominated by the health problems of a long-lived, aging population, one can imagine that studies that last 5, 10, or even 50 years can answer many of the key questions on which clinicians will look to researchers for guidance. Many patients are already put on powerful drugs in their 40s, 50s, and 60s that they will take for the rest of their lives. The very success of some cancer treatments is shifting attention from short-term survival to the long-term sequelae of treatment. For all these reasons, the era during which a genetic researcher simply needed a blood sample and a reliable diagnosis is passing.

Outcomes research is also creating new opportunities for a close integration of medicine and data-intensive biology. Cost constraints on health-care services—as well as an increasing appreciation of how often conventional medical wisdom is wrong—has led to a growing outcomes-research enterprise that barely existed a few decades ago. The requirements of outcomes researchers for access to uniform medical records of large patient populations are remarkably similar to those of molecularly oriented researchers.

MULTIPLE STAKEHOLDERS ARE READY FOR CHANGE

The tremendous recent progress in genetics, molecular biology, and information technology has been projected to lead to novel therapeutics and improved health-care outcomes with reduced overall health-care costs. However, there is little evidence that these benefits are accruing in mainstream medicine

(OECD 2011). Instead, health-care costs have steadily increased, and these increased costs have not necessarily translated into significantly better clinical outcomes (OECD 2011). This situation has created a "perfect storm" for a wide variety of stakeholders, including health-care providers, payers, regulators, patients, and drug developers. The economics of the present situation are not sustainable and demand change.

Clinical and basic researchers have learned that for their collective efforts to provide affordable improvements in health care, increased collaboration and coordination are required. Public–private collaborations are needed to combine longitudinal health outcomes data with new advances in technology and basic research. Such initiatives are essential to gain and apply the specific biological knowledge required to develop new approaches to treat and prevent disease. A dynamically evolving Knowledge Network of Disease would provide a framework in which a closer, more effective, relationship between clinical and basic researchers could thrive.

Nowhere is the need for change more evident and urgent than in the pharmaceutical and biotechnology industries. Despite a massive increase in the amount of genomic and molecular information available over the past decade, the number of effective new therapies developed each year has remained stable, while the cost of developing each successful therapy has increased dramatically (Munos 2009). While the new molecular technologies have identified a large number of novel drug targets, an inadequate biological understanding of these targets has resulted in an ever-increasing failure rate of expensive clinical trials (Arrowsmith 2011a,b). The present situation in drug development is not sustainable. The pharmaceutical and biotechnology industries are now leading proponents for developing public–private collaborations and consortia in which longitudinal clinical outcomes data can be combined with new molecular technology to develop the deep biological understanding needed to re-define disease based on biological mechanisms. Given the time scale on which private entities must seek return on investment, there is an increased willingness to regard much of this information as precompetitive. Hence, the information itself, and the costs of acquiring it, must be widely shared.

A major beneficiary of the proposed Knowledge Network of Disease and New Taxonomy would be what has been termed "precision medicine." In precision medicine, the ultimate end point is the selection of a subset of patients, with a common biological basis of disease, who are most likely to benefit from a drug or other treatment, such as a particular surgical procedure. Today, researchers look for relatively small differences between treated and untreated patients in trials that involve unselected patients, with little insight into the biological heterogeneity among the patients or their diseases. This approach requires a much larger number of patients, more time, and greater costs to assess the effectiveness of new therapies than would more targeted study designs. By using a precision-medicine approach to focus on those patients early in the drug-development

Box 2-4
Precision Medicine for Drug Development

A successful example of the precision medicine approach to drug development involves the drug Crizotinib, an inhibitor of the MET and ALK kinases, which began clinical development in a broad population of patients with lung cancer (Kwak et al. 2010). During the early stages of the initial Crizotinib clinical trial conducted by pharmaceutical industry scientists, an independent group of academic scientists published their discovery that a particular chromosomal translocation involving the gene encoding ALK drives tumor growth in a subset of non-small cell lung cancer patients (Soda et al. 2007). Access to this knowledge allowed the pharmaceutical industry scientists to modify their clinical trial to look specifically at a cohort of patients with this translocation, and the results were dramatic. For those patients who had the translocation, the median disease-free survival with Crizotinib was a year, compared to just a few months with the standard of care. Thus, even in a trial that involved only a small number of patients that were compared to historical controls, it was obvious that the drug was active. In contrast, in an unselected patient population, most patients did not benefit from this drug and it was unclear whether the drug had any activity.

(Crizotinib is expected to receive regulatory approval for treatment of ALK translocation-positive lung cancer within the next year.)

process who are most likely to be helped, fewer side effects and reduced costs are likely to ensue. In such studies, compliance will likely be better, treatment duration longer, and therapeutic benefits more obvious than is the case with traditional designs. Greater therapeutic differences could also result in more efficient regulatory approval, and faster adoption by physicians and payers.

As illustrated in Box 2-4, data sharing is essential to the development of precision medicine. Data sharing needs to occur across companies and across academic institutions to ensure that everyone benefits from fundamental biological knowledge. Institutions need to be convinced that they gain from openness. Broad engagement of a vast array of public and private stakeholders, including university scientists, regulators, health-care providers, payers, government, and perhaps most importantly the public at large, will be required to support and sustain the changes required for development of innovative new therapies that improve health outcomes based on the proposed Knowledge Network of Disease and associated New Taxonomy.

PUBLIC ATTITUDES TOWARD INFORMATION AND PRIVACY ARE IN FLUX

Genetic privacy was a central preoccupation during the early years of genomics, which led to implementation of stringent regulatory procedures to limit the use of genetic data in patient-oriented research (Andrews and Jaeger 1991). Many privacy-related issues—ranging from insurance coverage to employment discrimination, social stigmatization, and the simple desire to be left alone—are by no means resolved, although passage of the Genetic Information Nondiscrimination Act (GINA) alleviates many concerns about such discrimination (Hudson et al. 2008). During the ensuing years, the diffusion of the internet into every corner of our lives is driving massive changes in public attitudes toward privacy. Research studies of public attitudes reveal deep ambivalence about informational privacy. In the particular arena of genetic information and health records, members of focus groups typically grasp the broad social benefits of sharing data. A consistent theme is that people who contribute their own information to public databases want to be asked for permission, to have a clear explanation of how the data will be used, and to be treated as true partners in the research process (Damschroder et al. 2007; Trinidad et al. 2010; Haga and O'Daniel 2011). Although privacy concerns remain, there is little evidence that the public has the extreme sensitivity toward genetic data that many researchers anticipated 25 years ago.

THE PROPOSED KNOWLEDGE NETWORK OF DISEASE COULD CATALYZE CHANGES IN BIOLOGY, INFORMATION TECHNOLOGY, MEDICINE, AND SOCIETY

The powerful forces affecting basic biological research, information technology, clinical medicine, and public attitudes toward the privacy of health records and personal genetic information create an unprecedented opportunity to change how biomedical research is conducted and to improve health outcomes. The development of the proposed Knowledge Network of Disease and its associated New Taxonomy could take advantage of these forces to inspire revolutionary change. This Committee regards commitment to the development of these resources as a powerful unifying idea that could harness—and, to an appropriate degree, redirect—the creative energies of the key constituencies to achieve the full potential of biology to improve health outcomes.

3

What Would a Knowledge Network and New Taxonomy Look Like?

In the previous chapter, the Committee outlined the reasons it concluded that the time is right to develop a Knowledge Network of Disease and New Taxonomy. But what would these resources look like and what implications would they have for disease classification, basic research, clinical care, and the health-care system? This chapter describes the Committee's vision of a comprehensive Knowledge Network of Disease and New Taxonomy that would unite the biomedical-research, public-health, and health-care-delivery communities around the related goals of advancing our understanding of disease pathogenesis and improving health. The Committee envisions that the proposed resources would have several key features:

- They would drive development of a disease taxonomy that describes and defines diseases based on their intrinsic biology in addition to traditional physical "signs and symptoms".
- They would go beyond description and be directly linked to a deeper understanding of disease mechanisms, pathogenesis, and treatments.
- They would be highly dynamic, continuously incorporating newly emerging disease information.
- They would be based on an Information Commons that draws upon as much disease-related information, from as large a number of individual patients, as possible.
- Much of the data that would populate the Information Commons would be generated during the ordinary course of clinical care.

THE KNOWLEDGE NETWORK OF DISEASE
WOULD INCORPORATE MULTIPLE PARAMETERS
AND ENABLE A TAXONOMY HEAVILY ROOTED
IN THE INTRINSIC BIOLOGY OF DISEASE

Physical signs and symptoms are the overt manifestations of disease observed by physicians and patients. However, symptoms are not the best descriptors of disease. Symptoms are often non-specific and rarely identify a disease unambiguously. Physical signs and symptoms are generally also difficult to measure quantitatively. Furthermore, numerous diseases—including some of the most common ones such as cancer, cardiovascular disease, and HIV infection—are asymptomatic in early stages. Indeed, in a strict sense, all diseases are presumably asymptomatic for some "latent period" following the initiation of pathological processes. As a consequence, diagnosis based on traditional "signs and symptoms" alone carries the risk of missing opportunities for prevention, or early intervention can readily misdiagnose patients altogether. Even when histological analysis is performed, typically on tissue obtained after diseases become clinically evident, obtaining optimal diagnostic results can depend on supplementing standard histology with ancillary genetic or immunohistochemical testing to identify specific mutations or marker proteins.

Biology-based indicators of disease such as genetic mutations, marker-protein molecules, and other metabolites have the potential to be precise descriptors of disease. They can be measured accurately and precisely—be it in the form of a standardized biochemical assay or a genetic sequence—thus enabling comparison across datasets obtained from independent studies. Particularly when multiple molecular indicators are used in combination with conventional clinical, histological, and laboratory findings, they offer the opportunity for a more accurate and precise description and classification of disease.

Numerous molecularly-based disease markers are already available, and the number will grow rapidly in the future. Among the most prominent parameters of disease are an individual's:

- Genome
- Transcriptome
- Proteome
- Metabolome
- Lipidome
- Epigenome

As discussed in Chapter 2, it is increasingly feasible to obtain substantial information about these biological features for each individual patient. The cost of sequencing an individual's genome is rapidly dropping, and significant advances in the ability to globally and affordably characterize proteomes, metabolomes, lipidomes, epigenomes, and microbiomes of individual subjects will continue, creating the potential for an increasingly rich molecular characterization of individuals in the future. Eventually, it is likely that extensive molecular characterization of individuals will occur routinely as a normal part of health care—even prior to appearance of disease, thereby allowing the collection of data on both sick and healthy individuals on a scale vastly exceeding current practice. In addition to providing a new resource for research on disease processes, these data would provide a far more flexible and useful definition of the "normal" state, in all its diversity, than now exists. The ability to make such measurements on both non-affected tissues and in sites altered by disease would allow monitoring of the development and natural history of many disorders about which even the most basic information is presently unavailable.

THE INFORMATION COMMONS ON WHICH THE KNOWLEDGE NETWORK AND NEW TAXONOMY WOULD BE BASED WOULD INCORPORATE MUCH INFORMATION THAT CANNOT PRESENTLY BE DESCRIBED IN MOLECULAR TERMS

It is well recognized that health outcomes, disease phenotypes, and treatment response are determined by the individual and combined effects of various factors ranging from the molecular to the environmental (Collins 2004; IOM 2006; HealthyPeople.gov 2011). Gene-environment interactions have been implicated in a diverse group of diseases and pathological processes, including some psychological illnesses (Caspi et al. 2010), hypertension (Franks et al. 2004), tumor growth (J.B. Williams et al. 2009), HIV (Nunez et al. 2010), asthma (Chen et al. 2009), and cardiovascular reactivity (Williams et al. 2001; Snieder et al. 2002). Furthermore, the fact that numerous genome-wide association studies (GWASs) have revealed rather modest, albeit highly statistically significant, hazard ratios of disease risk highlights the need to investigate interactions among genetic and non-genetic factors to identify specific disease risk factors not found in conventional GWAS studies (Khoury and Wacholder 2009; Murcray et al. 2009; Cornelis et al 2010). Therefore, data added to the Information Commons should not be limited to molecular parameters as they are currently understood: patient-related data on environmental, behavioral, and socioeconomic factors will need to be considered as well in a thorough description of disease features[1] (see Box 3-1).

Despite the focus on the individual patient in the creation of the Information Commons, the Committee expects that the inclusion of patients from diverse populations coupled with the incorporation of various types of infor-

---

[1] As with all patient-related data in electronic medical records and contributed to the Information Commons, information in the exposome layer requires that attention be paid to data sharing, informed consent, and privacy issues; see discussion Chapter 4.

Box 3-1
The Exposome

The exposome is a characterization of both exogenous and endogenous exposures that can have differential effects on disease predisposition at various stages during a person's lifetime (Wild 2005; Rappaport 2011). The emerging science of exposomics is concerned with the application of innovative approaches to comprehensively measure a person's exposure events, from conception to death, and determine how those exposures relate to health and disease (CDC 2010; NAS 2010; Rappaport 2011). A long-range goal is to ascertain the combined effects of these exposures by assessing the biomarkers and diseases they influence.

In its broadest definition, the exposome encompasses all exposures—internal (such as the microbiome, described elsewhere in this report) and external—across the lifespan. Physical environment (e.g., occupational hazards, exposure to industrial and household pollutants, water quality, climate, altitude, air pollution, and living conditions (Smith et al. 2008; Klecka et al. 2010; Alexeeff et al. 2011; Brookhart et al. 2011; Cutts et al. 2011; Yorifuji et al. 2011; Zanobetti et al. 2011; McMichael and Lindgren 2011) and lifestyle and behavior (e.g., diet, physical activity, cultural practices, and use of addictive substances [DHHS 2010; Hu and Malik 2010; Arem et al. 2011]), are some of the more apparent exogenous exposures. However, the concept of the exposome extends beyond these factors to include social factors, such as socioeconomic status, quality of housing, neighborhood, social relationships, access to services, and experience of discrimination that can contribute to psychological stress, poor health, and health inequities (Epel et al. 2004; Krieger et al. 2005; IOM 2006; Cole et al. 2007; Unnatural Causes 2008; Bruce et al. 2009; Gravlee 2009; Williams and Mohammed 2009; Cardarelli et al. 2010; Kim et al. 2010; Pollack et al. 2010; CDC 2011; Karelina and DeVries 2011; Sternthal et al. 2011; WHO 2011).

Despite the many practical and methodological challenges in characterizing and measuring these variables, rigorous evaluation of human exposures is needed. By incorporating data derived from multi-level assessments, a Knowledge Network of Disease could lead to better understanding of the variables and mechanisms underlying disease and health disparities, thereby helping to reveal a truer picture of the ecology of human health and facilitating a more holistic approach to health promotion and disease prevention.

mation contained in the exposome will result in a Knowledge Network that could also inform the identification of population-level interventions and the improvement of population health. For example, a better understanding of the impact of a sedentary lifestyle at the molecular level could conceivably facilitate the development of new approaches to physical education in early childhood. In addition, findings from the Knowledge Network and the New Taxonomy could reveal yet unidentified behavioral, social, and environmental factors that are associated with particular diseases or subclassifications of diseases in certain populations and are amenable to public health interventions.

The Healthy People 2020 Initiative (Healthy People.gov. 2011) emphasizes an ecological approach to disease prevention and health promotion that focuses on both individual-level and population-level determinants of health and interventions. While molecular variables are often more easily measured and more directly tied to disease outcomes, if the modifiable factors that have contributed to the signature are known, we will be better able to prevent disease and to phenotype, genotype, and treat patients.

Asthma illustrates the interplay of social, behavioral, environmental, and genetic factors in disease classification. It is estimated that various types of asthma affect more than 300 million people worldwide. The term "asthma" is now used to refer to a set of "signs and symptoms" including reversible airway narrowing ("wheezing"), airway inflammation and remodeling, and airway hyper-reactivity. These various signs and symptoms likely reflect distinct etiologies in different patients. Many subjects with asthma have an allergic component, while in other cases, no clear allergic contributor can be defined (Hill et al. 2011; Lee et al. 2011). In some patients, asthma attacks are precipitated by exercise or aspirin (Cheong et al. 2011). Some patients, particularly those with severe asthma, may be resistant to treatment with corticosteroids (Searing et al. 2010). This phenomenological approach to asthma diagnosis has led to a plethora of asthma subtypes such as "allergic asthma," "exercise-induced asthma," and "steroid-resistant asthma" that may be clinically useful but provide little insight into underlying etiologies.

Over the years, linkage-analysis, candidate-gene, and genome-wide-association approaches have been applied to the study of the genetic underpinnings of asthma, leading to the identification of several associated genes and subphenotypes (Lee et al. 2011). However, these findings still leave most of the genetic influences of asthma unexplained (Li et al. 2010; Moffatt et al. 2010). Moreover, pediatric asthma research, in particular, has focused on a broad range of social and environmental, as well as genetic, contributors to the increased prevalence and severity of illness (Hill et al. 2011). Since the burden of asthma disproportionately affects children living in socioeconomically disadvantaged neighborhoods (D.R. Williams et al. 2009; Quinn et al. 2010), asthma may prove useful as a model for testing the Knowledge Network's value in attaining a broader and deeper understanding of disease and health, in both the clinical and public-health policy domains. A knowledge-network-derived-taxonomy based on the biology of disease may help to divide patients with asthma—as well as many other diseases—into subtypes in which the different etiologies of the disorder can be better understood, and for which appropriate, subtype-specific approaches to treatment and prevention can be devised and tested.

THE PROPOSED KNOWLEDGE NETWORK OF DISEASE WOULD INCLUDE INFORMATION ABOUT PATHOGENS AND OTHER MICROBES

Particularly because of advances in genomics, the proposed Knowledge Network of Disease has unprecedented potential to incorporate information about disease-causing and disease-associated microbial agents. Thousands of microbial genomes have been sequenced, providing a wealth of data on pathogenic and non-pathogenic organisms, and there has been an associated renaissance in studies of the molecular mechanisms of host-pathogen interactions. In parallel with these advances in microbiology, the analysis of human-genome sequences is enhancing the understanding of host responses and variation in individual susceptibility to microbial pathogens and infectious diseases. Today, sequence data, combined with other biochemical and microbiological information, are being used to understand microbial contribution to health, improve detection of pathogens, diagnose infectious diseases, and identify potential new targets for novel drugs and vaccines. In addition, comparing the sequences of different strains, species, and clinical isolates is crucial for identifying genetic polymorphisms that correlate with phenotypes such as drug resistance, morbidity, and infectivity. Combining this information with the molecular signature of the host will provide a more complete picture of an individual's diseases allowing custom-tailoring of therapeutic interventions.

THE PROPOSED KNOWLEDGE NETWORK OF DISEASE WOULD GO BEYOND DESCRIPTION

A Knowledge Network of Disease would aspire to go far beyond disease description. It would seek to provide a unifying framework within which basic biology, clinical research, and patient care could co-evolve. The scope of the Knowledge Network's influence would encompass:

Disease classification. The use of multiple molecular-based parameters to characterize disease may lead to more accurate and finer-grained classification of disease (see Box 3-2). Disease classification is not merely an academic exercise: more nuanced diagnostic accuracy and ability to recognize disease subtypes would undoubtedly have important therapeutic consequences, allowing treatment regimes to be customized based on the precise molecular features of a patient's disease.

Disease-mechanism discovery. A Knowledge Network in which diseases are increasingly understood and defined in terms of molecular pathways has the potential to accelerate discovery of underlying disease mechanisms. In a molecularly-based Knowledge Network, a researcher could readily compare the

---

Box 3-2
Distinguishing Disease Types

Recent progress in the classification of lymphomas illustrates how a Knowledge Network could help distinguish diseases or disease states with similar symptoms and clinical presentations. Gene-expression profiling led to the discovery that B-cell lymphomas comprise two distinct subtypes of disease with different driver mutations and different prognoses (Alizadeh et al. 2000; Sweetenham 2011). One subtype bears a gene-expression profile similar to germinal center B-cells and has a good prognosis, while a second subtype bears a gene-expression profile similar to activated B-cells and has a poor prognosis. Recognition of these biological and clinical differences between subtypes of B-cell lymphomas makes it possible to predict patient prognosis more accurately and guide treatment decisions.

Similarly, leukemias are also now categorized based on differences in driver mutations, revealing subtypes with different prognoses and responses to particular treatment approaches. Acute myeloid leukemias with FLT3/ITD mutations have a poorer prognosis than acute myeloid leukemias with a normal FLT3 gene (Kiyoi et al. 1999; Kottaridis et al. 2001). As a consequence, patients bearing FLT3/ITD mutations are more likely to receive allogenic bone-marrow transplants or be offered experimental therapy with FTLs kinase inhibitors, while patients who do not have FLT3/ITD mutations are more likely to be treated only with chemotherapy. These are two of many known examples in which molecular data have been used to distinguish subtypes of malignancies with different prognoses and that benefit from different treatments. The proposed Knowledge Network of Disease could be expected to lead to many more insights of this type. By allowing any researcher to carry out analyses of this type on large numbers of patients, tracked over long periods of time, it is likely that insights such as the clinical relevance of FLT3 mutations in leukemia could be achieved for many other cancers and in situations where tumor behavior depends on a more complex interplay of influences.

---

molecular fingerprint (such as one defined by the transcriptome or proteome) of a disease with an unknown pathogenic mechanism to the information available for better understood diseases. Similarities between the molecular profiles of diseases with known and unknown pathogenic mechanisms might point directly to shared disease mechanisms, or at least serve as a starting point for directed molecular interrogation of cellular pathways likely to be involved in the pathogenesis of both diseases.

Disease detection and diagnosis. A Knowledge Network that integrates data from many different levels of disease determinants collected from individual subjects over time may reveal new opportunities for detection and early diagnosis. The availability of information on a multitude of diverse diseases should facilitate epidemiological research to identify novel diagnostic markers based on correlations among diverse datasets (including clinical, social, economic, environmental, and lifestyle factors) and disease incidence, treatment decisions, and outcomes. In some instances, these advances would follow from the new insights into pathogenic mechanisms discussed above. The most robust early-detection tests—for example, assessment of an asymptomatic patient's HIV status—are based on a clear understanding of pathogenic mechanism. In other cases, however, molecular profiles may prove sufficiently predictive of a patient's future health to have substantial clinical utility long before the mechanistic rationale of the correlation is understood.

Disease predisposition. A Knowledge Network of Disease that links information from many levels of disease determinants, from genetic to environment and lifestyle, will improve our ability to predict and survey for diseases. Following outcomes in individual patients over time will allow the prognostic value of molecular-based classifications to be tested and, ideally, verified. Multi-parameter data across the entire spectrum of disease will become available. Obviously, the clinical utility of identifying disease predispositions depends on the availability of interventions that would either prevent or delay onset of disease or perhaps ameliorate disease severity.

Disease treatment. The ultimate goal of most clinical research is to improve disease treatments and health outcomes. There are many ways in which a Knowledge Network of Disease and its derived taxonomy may be expected to impact disease treatment and to contribute to improved health outcomes for patients. Accurate diagnosis is the foundation of all medical interventions. As many of the examples already discussed illustrate, finer-grained diagnoses often are the key to choosing optimal treatments. In some instances, a molecularly informed disease classification offers improved options for disease prevention or management even when different disease subtypes are treated identically (see Box 3-3). A Knowledge Network that integrates data from multiple levels of disease determinants will also facilitate the development of new therapies by identifying new therapeutic targets and may suggest off-label use of existing drugs. In other cases, the identification of links between environmental factors or lifestyle choices and disease incidence may make it possible to reduce disease incidence by lifestyle interventions.

Importantly, as discussed below, the Committee believes the Knowledge Network and its underlying Information Commons would enable the discovery of improved treatments by providing a powerful new research resource that would bring together researchers with diverse skills and integrate knowledge about disease processes in an unprecedented way. Indeed, it is quite possible that the transition to a modernized "discovery model" in which disease data generated during the course of normal health care and analyzed by a diverse set

> **Box 3-3**
> **Information to Guide Treatment Decisions**
>
> The example of a patient such as Patient 1 with breast cancer, described in the Introduction, illustrates the potential of a Knowledge Network of Disease to provide patients with valuable information even when there is no difference in treatment for different diseases subtypes (e.g., sporadic vs. *BRCA1/2*-associated breast cancer). While mutations in the tumor-suppressor genes *BRCA1* and *BRCA2* strongly predispose women to breast and ovarian cancer, the extent to which particular germline mutations in these genes increase cancer risk often remains uncertain (Gayther et al. 1995). Consequently, patients and physicians must currently make decisions about whether to undertake more intensive cancer surveillance (for example, by breast magnetic resonance imaging or vaginal ultrasound) without being able clearly to assess the risks and benefits of such increased screening and the anxiety and potential morbidity that arises from inevitable false positives. Furthermore, some patients elect to undergo prophylactic mastectomies or oophorectomies without definitive information about the extent to which these drastic procedures actually would reduce their cancer risk.
>
> Studies attempting to quantify these risks have largely focused on particular ethnic groups in which a limited set of mutations occur at high enough frequencies to allow reliable conclusions from analyses carried out on a practical scale. If *BRCA1/2* genotypes and health histories could be compared across the large datasets currently segregated among different health-care organizations, it would become possible to assess accurately cancer risks for people with different mutations and genetic backgrounds. Such data would allow more rational recommendations regarding risk-reduction strategies, thereby creating enormous value for individual patients, health-care providers, and payers, by making it possible to avoid unnecessary screening and treatment while reducing cancer incidence and promoting early detection.

of researchers would ultimately prove to be a Knowledge Network of Disease's greatest legacy for biomedical research.

Drug development. Molecular similarities among seemingly unrelated diseases would also be of direct relevance to drug discovery as it would lead to targeted investigation of disease-relevant pathways that are shared between molecularly related diseases. In addition, ongoing access to molecular profiles and health histories of large numbers of patients taking already-approved drugs would undoubtedly lead to improved drug safety by allowing identification of individuals at higher-than-normal risk of adverse drug reactions. Indeed, our limited understanding of—and lack of a robust system for studying—rare adverse reactions is a major barrier to the introduction of new drugs in our increasingly risk-aversive and litigious society.

Health disparities. Major disparities in the health profiles of different "racial", ethnic, and socio-economic groups within our diverse society have proven discouragingly refractory to amelioration. As discussed above, it is quite likely that key contributors to these disparities can be most effectively addressed through public-health measures and other public policies that have little to do with the molecular basis of disease, at least as we presently understand it. However, the Committee regards the Information Commons and Knowledge Network of Disease, as potentially powerful tools for understanding and addressing health disparities because they would be informed by data on the environmental and social factors that influence the health of individual patients. For the first time, these resources would bring together, in the same place, molecular profiles, health histories, and data on the many determinants of health and disease, thereby optimizing the ability to decipher the mechanisms through which exogenous factors give rise to endogenous, biological inputs, directly affecting health. Researchers and policy makers would then be better able to sort out the full diversity of possible reasons for observed individual and group differences in health and to devise effective strategies to prevent and combat them.

A HIERARCHY OF LARGE DATASETS WOULD BE THE FOUNDATION OF THE KNOWLEDGE NETWORK OF DISEASE AND ITS PRACTICAL APPLICATIONS

The establishment of a Knowledge Network, and its research and clinical applications, would depend on the availability of a hierarchy of large, well-integrated datasets describing what we know about human disease. These datasets would establish the foundation for the New Taxonomy and many other basic and applied activities throughout the health-care system. The Information Commons would contain the raw information about individual patients from which meaningful links and relationships could be derived. Recognizing that the Knowledge Network would need to be informed by vast amounts of information external to the network itself, the Committee envisions the need for substantial research in medical informatics directed at all steps of the creation and curation of the network, and, equally importantly, its use by individuals with diverse backgrounds and goals. The creation of the Knowledge Network and its underlying Information Commons would enable the continuous compilation and analysis of molecular, environmental, behavioral, social, and clinical data in a dynamic, shared platform. Such an information platform would need to be accessible by users across the entire spectrum of research and clinical care, including payers. Data would be continuously deposited by the research community and extracted directly from the medical records of participating patients. The roles of the different datasets in this information resource are schematized in Figure 3-1.

The precise structures of both the Information Commons and Knowledge Network of Disease remain to be determined and would be informed by pilot studies, as discussed in Chapter 4. However, given its purpose, the Committee envisions the Information Commons as (see also Figure 1-2):

Multilayered. Given the inclusion of multiple parameters ranging from genomic to environmentally modulated disease factors, the Information Commons would likely have a multi-layered structure with each layer containing the information for one disease parameter, such as "signs and symptoms", genetic mutations, epigenetic patterns, metabolic characteristics, or other risk factors (including social, behavioral, and environmental influences).

Individual-centric. The Information Commons should register all measurements with respect to individuals so that the multitude of influences on pathophysiological states can be viewed at scales that span all the way from the molecular to the social level. Only in this way could, for example, individual environmental exposures be matched to individual changes in molecular profiles. These data would need to be stored in an escrowed, encrypted depository that allows graded release of data depending on the questions asked, the access level of the individual making the inquiry, and other parameters that would undoubtedly emerge in the course of pilot studies. The Committee realizes that this is a radical approach and intense public education and outreach about the value of the Information Commons to the progress of medicine would be essential to harness informed volunteerism, the support of disease-specific advocacy groups, and the engagement of other stakeholders. The Committee regards careful handling of policies to ensure privacy as the central issue in its entire vision of the Information Commons, the Knowledge Network of Disease, and the New Taxonomy. Hence, this topic is discussed in more detail in Chapter 4.

The Knowledge Network of Disease, created by integrating data in the Information Commons with fundamental biological knowledge, drawn from the biomedical literature and existing community databases such as GenBank, would be the centerpiece of the informational resources underlying the New Taxonomy. The Committee envisions this network as:

Highly inter-connected. In order to extract relationship information between multiple parameters—for example, the transcriptome and the exposome—the multiple data layers must be inter-connected (see Figure 3-1). Ideally, each information layer would be connected to every other layer: thus, "signs and symptoms" would be linked to mutations, mutations to metabolic defects, exposome

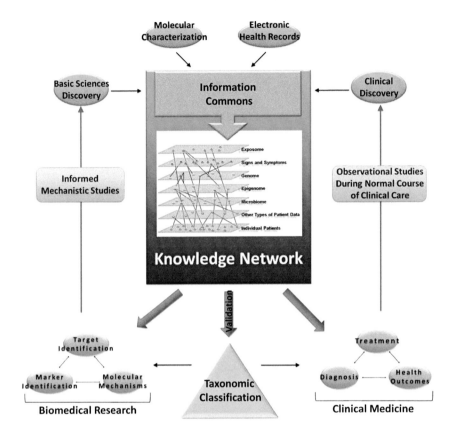

FIGURE 3-1 Building a biomedical Knowledge Network for basic discovery and Medicine.

At the center of a comprehensive biomedical information network is an Information Commons that contains current disease information linked to individual patients and is continuously updated by a wide set of new data emerging though observational studies during the course of normal health care. The data in the Information Commons and Knowledge Network serve three purposes: (1) they provide the basis to generate a dynamic, adaptive system that informs taxonomic classification of disease; (2) they provide the foundation for novel clinical approaches (diagnostics, treatments, strategies), and (3) they provide a resource for basic discovery. Validated findings that emerge from the Knowledge Network, such as those which define new diseases or subtypes of diseases that are clinically relevant (e.g., which have implications for patient prognosis or therapy) would be incorporated into the New Taxonomy to improve diagnosis (i.e., disease classification) and treatment. The fine-grained nature of the taxonomic classification would aid in clinical decision-making by more accurately defining disease.

SOURCE: Committee on A Framework for Developing a New Taxonomy of Disease.

to the epigenome, and so forth. The links could be one-to-one but most commonly would be many-to-one, and one-to-many (e.g., particular signs and symptoms arise when other parameters fall into many otherwise unrelated clusters). The interrelationships among such features within and between the layers could be characterized through a variety of representations that attempt to extract meaning from the Information Commons. For example, distinct transcriptomes may define several types of B-cell lymphomas. Meanwhile, different types of lymphomas, defined by transcriptome analysis, may have distinct metabolomic profiles. The similarities of multiple diseases could be discerned either from relationships among the networks of individual parameters (e.g., transcriptomes of multiple B-cell lymphomas) or from common patterns that emerge once multiple parameters are combined.

Flexible. A highly inter-connected Knowledge Network would link multiple individual networks of parameters in a flexible way. A user could chose to interrogate only a small part of the network by limiting his or her analysis to a single information layer, or even a small portion of this layer; alternatively, a user could interrogate the complex interrelationship of multiple parameters. High flexibility ensures easy cross-comparison and cross-correlation of any desired dataset, making it a versatile tool for a wide spectrum of applications ranging from basic research to clinical studies and healthy system administration.

Widely accessible. The Knowledge Network would need to be accessible and usable by a wide range of stakeholders from basic scientists to clinicians, health-care workers, and the public. Furthermore, the available information would need to be mineable in ways that are custom-tailored to the needs of different users, possibly by implementation of purpose-specific user interfaces.

While the Committee agreed upon the generalities listed above and illustrated in Figure 3-1 about the Information Commons and Knowledge Network —and their relationship to a New Taxonomy— specifics of implementation such as the detailed design of the Information Commons, the information technology platforms used to create it, questions about where key infrastructure should be physically housed, who would oversee it, and how the Information Commons would be financed, were considered beyond the scope of the Committee's charge in a framework study. Nonetheless, dramatic developments in the fields of medical information technology—and other developments discussed in Chapter 2—give the Committee confidence that the creation and implementation of this ambitious and novel infrastructure is a feasible goal.

THE PROPOSED KNOWLEDGE NETWORK WOULD FUNDAMENTALLY DIFFER FROM CURRENT BIOMEDICAL INFORMATION SYSTEMS

Immense progress has been made during the past 25 years in organizing our knowledge of basic biology, health, and disease, even as many components of this knowledge base have grown super-exponentially. The National Library of Medicine and its National Center for Biotechnology Information division (NCBI), created in 1988, maintains the closest current counterpart to the information infrastructure that the Committee envisions. The NCBI maintains a vast array of information about basic biology, health, and disease—ranging from the PubMed system for indexing the biomedical literature to GenBank, the primary depository for DNA-sequence data—and its databases are queried daily by nearly anyone involved in biomedical research. So, what is the difference between the Committee's vision of the Information Commons and Knowledge Network of Disease and reasonable extrapolations of what the NCBI has already accomplished?

The key difference is that the Information Commons, which would underlie the other databases, would be "individual-centric." The various databanks curated by NCBI generally only contain a single disease parameter and even if multiple pieces of information from an individual make it into multiple databanks—say a breast cancer patient's transcriptome stored in the GeneOmnibus database of published microarray data and information about her chromosome translocations in the Cancer Chromosome databank—they are not linked between databases. An independent researcher, who was not involved in the study that contributed these entries, has no way of knowing that they are from the same individual. As a consequence, relationships between multiple parameters that determine disease status in a given individual are impossible to extract. However, motivated by the recent proliferation of GWAS studies, NCBI has developed an individual-centric database, dbGap (the database of Genotypes and Phenotypes). This database was "developed to archive and distribute the results of studies that have investigated the interaction of genotype and phenotype" (NCBI 2011b). The Committee considers NCBI's success in doing so—despite severe current constraints on the sharing of phenotypic information about individuals—as evidence that the obstacles to creating an Information Commons can be overcome. This issue is discussed in more detail in Chapter 4. However, the important point is that little of the NCBI's vast current store of information could, even in principle, be organized along the lines suggested for the Information Commons. This information was not collected in a way that allows the individual to be the central organizing principle, and no amount of redesign of the inter-connections between different entries in the current system could achieve the goals the Committee has outlined.

The Committee would like to emphasize the novelty and power of an

Information Commons that is "individual-centric." As discussed in Chapter 2, a useful analogy is geographical information systems (GISs) such as Google Maps (see Figure 1-2). Following public access to the Global Positioning System (GPS) and dramatic improvements in database technology in many ways analogous to the driving forces current advances in data generation and handling in biomedicine, it became apparent to many users of geographically indexed information that a surprisingly high portion of the world's information could be organized around GPS coordinates. Like the proposed Information Commons, GISs are layered data structures that inter-connect vast amounts of information and can be mined for information that is not readily apparent in the primary GPS of an object. For example, given the coordinates of a large number of, say, backyard barbecue grills, one can suddenly overlay a vast amount of socio-economic, ethnic, climatological, and other data on what—at the start of the investigation—appeared a peculiar, anecdotal inquiry. In some respects, this approach is counter-intuitive. The GPS coordinates of someone's backyard barbecue grill may appear to take one away from useful generalizations about grills: it reveals more detail than one might want to know about an individual grill without laying any obvious foundations for developing an integrated perspective on the cultural practice of backyard-barbecuing. However, it is the precise GPS coordinates of an individual grill that are the key to inter-connecting whatever has been learned about this particular grill to a larger world of information.

Despite significant challenges to constructing an individual-centric Information Commons, the Committee concluded that this is a realistic undertaking and would be essential to the success of the Knowledge-Network/New Taxonomy initiative. *The Committee is of the opinion that "precision medicine," designed to provide the best accessible care for each individual, is not achievable without a massive reorientation of the information systems on which researchers and health-care providers depend: these systems, like the medicine they aspire to support, must be individualized.* Generalizations must be built up from information on large numbers of individuals. Efforts to reverse this process will fail since indispensable information is lost when molecular profiles, data on other aspects of an individual's circumstances, and health histories are abstracted away from the individual at the very beginning of investigations into the determinants of health and disease.

A KNOWLEDGE NETWORK OF DISEASE
WOULD CONTINUOUSLY EVOLVE

Although knowledge of disease, and particularly molecular mechanisms of pathogenesis, is still limited, the pace of progress has never been greater. New insights into the biology of disease are emerging rapidly from a wealth of molecular approaches, as well as from new insights into the importance of environmental factors. However, the system for updating current disease taxonomies, at intervals of many years does not permit the rapid incorporation of new information, thereby contributing to the delayed introduction of advances that have the potential, over time, to guide mainstream practice. The individual-centric nature of an Information Commons is an important means of ensuring that the data underlying the Knowledge Network, and its derived taxonomy, would be constantly updated. As participating patients undergo new tests and treatments, associated information would enter the Information Commons and, on the basis of these data, the taxonomies, such as the ICD, could be updated continuously. Such a dynamic system would not only accept new inputs for established disease parameters, it would also accommodate new types of information generated by newly developed technologies to identify, acquire, measure, and analyze new biological features of disease.

THE NEW TAXONOMY WOULD REQUIRE
CONTINUOUS VALIDATION

Bad information is worse than no information. A key feature of a clinically useful taxonomy is the requirement for a validation system. The logic of the classification scheme, and especially its utility for practical applications, needs to be carefully and continuously tested. This is particularly important when patients and clinicians use the New Taxonomy to inform clinical decisions. The New Taxonomy should be routinely tested to provide all stakeholders with data indicating the extent to which decisions guided by it can be made with confidence. Clearly, some patients and clinicians will be more comfortable than others with making decisions that are based on clinical intuition rather than proven evidence. However, a physician should be able to interrogate the Knowledge Network that underlies the New Taxonomy to learn whether others have had to make a similar decision, and, if so, what the consequences were. For example, if a drug has been introduced to target a particular driver mutation in a cancer, a physician needs to know whether or not rigorous clinical testing has determined that the drug is safe and effective. Is the drug effective only in some patients who can be identified in some way, such as by analyzing variants of genes that affect cell growth or drug metabolism? Similarly, if a laboratory test is considered to be a candidate predictor for the later development of disease, has that hypothesis been rigorously validated? Is the candidate test valid in some patient groups but not others? Whether a given test is used to identify predictors of disease or the existence of disease, the test result must be interpreted in the context of knowledge about the "normal range" of results. This requirement is not a trivial consideration, especially for tests based on integration of vast amounts of data, such as the genome, transcriptome, and metabolome of the patient. Even with a conventional sequencing test, it is often difficult to ascertain with certainty whether a sequence change is disease-causing or insignificant. This dilemma is multiplied many times over for genome-level testing. Some initial results from whole-human-genome-sequencing data indicate the scale of this problem: most individuals have dozens to hundreds of sequence variants that are readily recognizable, on biochemical grounds, as potentially pathogenic: examples include variants that cause premature-protein truncation or loss of normal stop codons (Ge et al. 2009; Pelak et al. 2010)—yet the clinical significance of nearly all such variants remains obscure. Defining and continuously refining our understanding of the normal "reference range" for such tests would require being able to access and effectively analyze biological and other relevant clinical data derived from large and ethnically diverse populations. Ultimately, the Knowledge Network that underlies the New Taxonomy will make it possible to develop decision-support tools that synthesize information and alert health-care providers to all validated insights that emerge from the Knowledge Network and that are relevant to clinical decisions under consideration.

THE NEW TAXONOMY WOULD DEVELOP IN PARALLEL WITH THE CONTINUED USE OF CURRENT TAXONOMIES

Existing disease taxonomies, such as ICD, clearly have utility and are likely to continue to be employed throughout the health-care system far into the future. The organizational and financial costs of systematically replacing these systems would be substantial. Moreover, as noted above, those responsible for revision of the ICD taxonomy are actively engaged in incorporating molecular characteristics of disease into that system. Hence, it is quite possible that the New Taxonomy could ultimately subsume the ICD system, with the latter comprising the most rigorously validated subset of disease classifications. Such issues must be addressed but, given the magnitude of the tasks associated with launching the creation of the Information Commons and the Knowledge Network of Disease, and seeing it through its formative stages, their consideration can safely be postponed for many years.

THE PROPOSED INFORMATIONAL INFRASTRUCTURE WOULD HAVE GLOBAL HEALTH IMPACT

A Knowledge Network of Disease should ultimately provide global benefits. Inevitably, the Knowledge Network initially would be devised primarily through data acquired, placed in the Information Commons, and analyzed by researchers and medical institutions in developed countries. However, a comprehensive and fully developed Knowledge Network of Disease must include the many diseases, including infectious diseases and disorders linked to geographically limited environmental exposures that are endemic in low- and middle-income settings throughout the world. Therefore, the Knowledge Network effort should be extended to include analysis of data derived in these settings.

Improved precision in defining disease is of particular importance in regions of the world with under-developed health-care systems. Disease misdiagnosis in such settings has contributed to the improper use of therapy and the establishment of widespread drug resistance among disease-causing infectious agents. Malaria is one disease where misdiagnosis is common with dramatic consequences and costs (D'Acremont et al. 2009). In general, patients presenting with fever in regions where malaria is endemic are administered anti-malarial treatment without direct evidence that the patient actually has malaria. In part, this practice is due to limited resources—the state-of-the-art diagnostic test in most areas is a microscopy-based blood-smear diagnosis, which requires expert training. The lack of adequate point-of-care diagnostic tests to ascertain whether the patient has malaria represents a significant impediment to the selection of appropriate targeted therapy. As a consequence, major efforts are under way to develop molecular diagnostics for malaria and other major killers such as tubercuolosis (Boehme et al. 2010; Small and Pai 2010). Ultimately, such diagnostics will need to include tests that differentiate among various disease agents and also take into account genetic or molecular markers in the host that influence host responses to the infection or potential treatments. A globally relevant Information Commons and Knowledge Network could be useful in facilitating this process—for example, to distinguish between malaria caused by *Plasmodium falciparum* versus *Plasmodium vivax*, which are susceptible to different anti-malarial drugs (malERA Consultative Group on Diagnoses and Diagnostics 2011). The Knowledge Network and its associated taxonomy should not be designed exclusively to meet the needs of countries with advanced medical systems. Indeed, the individual-centric character of the Information Commons—and the inclusion of available data about contributing individuals, including information about where and in what circumstances they live—offers an unprecedented path toward a Knowledge Network of Disease that can meet global needs for health care and disease prevention.

4

How Do We Get There?

After reaching consensus on the need for a New Taxonomy, the Committee deliberated extensively on the question "How do we get there?" In this context, "there" refers to successful creation of a system for acquiring and analyzing information relating the molecular profiles and health histories of large numbers of individuals. In Chapter 3, we describe the properties we would expect a Knowledge Network of Disease and the New Taxonomy to have and the type of Information Commons that would be needed to create them. However, we also emphasized that these resources will forever remain "works in progress." As information technology, basic science, health research, and medicine undergo successive waves of change, both the content and structure of the New Taxonomy and Information Commons are expected to evolve, likely in directions that are presently impossible to envision. Consider, by analogy, early attempts to conceptualize the world-wide web compared to the use of the internet today. The Committee's view is that we presently lack the infrastructure required to produce a dramatically improved disease taxonomy. Rather, we propose a path forward to develop the infrastructure and research system needed to create the Knowledge Network of Disease that we believe would be an essential underpinning of a molecularly-based taxonomy. We also address the sustainability of this initiative. Just as public leadership and investment played essential roles in bringing the world-wide web into existence, we believe such investment will be critical if we are to achieve a grand synthesis of data-intensive biology and medicine. However, we also recognize that, just as the world-wide web needed to pay its own way before it could truly flourish, the Knowledge Network and its underlying Information Commons will need to do the same.

The Committee believes that initiatives will be required in three areas to exploit the wealth of information now emerging on molecular mechanisms of disease by creating a dynamic and comprehensive, yet practical and widely-used, Knowledge Network:

1. *Design of appropriate strategies to collect and integrate disease-relevant information.* The Information Commons would be developed by linking molecular data to patient information on a massive scale. Creating a system for establishing this linkage for increasing numbers of individuals—and making the resulting data widely available to researchers—is the key step in moving toward a Knowledge Network and New Taxonomy. Such coupled data can be generated in several ways—including the modest-scale, targeted molecular studies on patient materials that dominate current practice. However, the most direct and effective discovery paradigm involves observational studies that seek to relate molecular data to complete patient medical records available as by-products of routine health care. Effective follow-up of the most promising hypotheses generated through such studies will require laboratory-based biological investigations designed to seek explanations at the biochemical or physiological levels.

2. *Implementation of pilot studies to establish a practical framework to discover relationships between and among molecular and other patient-specific data, patient diagnoses, and clinical outcomes.* The new discovery model will involve the mining of large sets of patient data acquired during the ordinary course of health care. This is a novel, largely untested discovery approach. Pilot studies designed to identify and overcome obstacles to successful implementation of this approach will be required before a set of "best practices" can emerge.

3. *Gradual elimination of institutional, cultural, and regulatory barriers to widespread sharing of the molecular profiles and health histories of individuals, while still protecting patients' rights.* The sharing of data about individual patients among multiple parties—including patients, physicians, insurance companies, the pharmaceutical industry, and academic research groups—will be essential. Current policies on consent, confidentiality, data protection and ownership, health cost reimbursement, and intellectual-property will need to be modified to ensure the free flow of research data between all stakeholders without compromising patient interests.

A NEW DISCOVERY MODEL FOR DISEASE RESEARCH

The current model for relating molecular data to diagnoses and clinical outcomes typically involves abstracting clinical data for a modest number of patients from a clinical to a research setting, then attempting to draw correlations between the abstracted clinical data and molecular data such as genetic polymorphisms, gene-expression levels, and metabolomic profiles. When discoveries are judged definitive and potentially useful, an effort is made to return this information to the clinical setting—for example, as a genetic or genomic diagnostic test. This model creates a large gulf between the point of discovery and the point of care with many opportunities for mis- and even non-communication between key stakeholders. For example, there have been approximately ten times more genome-wide association studies (GWASs) performed on individuals of European ancestry than other groups (Need and Goldstein 2009). The current model also fails to exploit the wealth of molecular data that are likely to be generated routinely in the future as personalized genomics and perhaps other personalized "omics" become routine in clinical settings. Perhaps most seriously, the current discovery model offers no path toward economically sustainable integration of data-intensive biology with medicine.

The Committee views it as both desirable and ultimately inevitable that this discovery model be fundamentally transformed. Instead of moving clinical data and patient samples to research groups to allow analysis, the molecular data of patients should instead be directly available to researchers and health-care providers. The Committee recognizes that this is a radical departure from current practice and one that faces significant challenges, nonetheless, because we believe this new discovery model would have dramatic benefits, we believe that aggressive steps should be taken to implement it.

The changes in science, information technology, medicine and social attitudes—as discussed in Chapter 2—provides the opportunity to implement this model. Indeed, there are concrete instances of research initiatives already underway that substantiate the Committee's belief that a special effort to implement its core recommendations can be achieved. In addition to the eMERGE Consortium discussed in Chapter 2, an excellent example is a collaboration between Kaiser-Permanente Northern California and the University of California at San Francisco (UCSF). Kaiser members were asked to participate in a study that would allow genetic and other molecular data to be compared with their full electronic health records. The study has faced major hurdles, and required more than ten years to progress from its conceptualization to large-scale acquisition of genetic data. A pivotal challenge was to build trust between Kaiser's members, management, and oversight groups such as the relevant Institutional Review Boards. While all parties recognized it was essential that the Kaiser members who were being asked to "opt in" to the research study be fully aware of its aims, the outreach infrastructure required to educate members had to be created nearly from scratch. A second major challenge was acquiring funding to cover the cost of generating extensive molecular data that lacked direct and immediate relevance to patient care—a responsibility that Kaiser itself could not be expected to take on given the pressure to constrain health-care costs. Moreover, changing perceptions about what constitutes appropriate informed consent required costly and time-consuming reconsenting of the participants.

Nonetheless, the ability of committed investigators—working within strongly supportive institutions—to overcome these obstacles has been impressive: nearly 200,000 Kaiser members have joined the study and large-scale data collection is now underway.

The pioneering UCSF-Kaiser study makes clear that a discovery model based on direct use of patient data is possible, even as its implementation faces significant hurdles. In order to address and resolve these hurdles, the Committee envisions the design of several targeted pilot studies. These studies would probe key aspects of this new research paradigm and demonstrate to healthcare providers the value of a molecularly informed taxonomy of disease. By demonstrating value for patients, the pilot studies will seek to lay the groundwork for a sustainable discovery model in which relevant clinically validated molecular data are routinely generated at the "point of care" because they meet the commonly accepted risk-benefit criteria that apply to all clinical test results.

PILOT STUDIES SHOULD DRAW UPON OBSERVATIONAL STUDIES

As emphasized above, the Committee believes that much of the initial work necessary to develop the Information Commons should take the form of observational studies. In this context, what we mean by observational studies is that, although molecular and other patient-specific data would be collected from individuals in the normal course of health care, no changes in the treatment of the individuals would be contingent on the data collected. This approach to discovery is already in use today, although most current initiatives draw in a very limited range of clinical data. Notably, many GWASs have compared the genetic make-ups of individuals who receive a diagnosis of a disease to those who do not (McCarthy et al. 2008). For example, GWASs comparing individuals with and without a diagnosis of Crohn's disease securely identified a number of gene variants that implicate autophagy in the pathophysiology of Crohn's disease while similar comparisons for Age-Related Macular Degeneration implicated complement factor H (McCarthy et al. 2008; Ryu et al. 2010). In other instances, clinically relevant genotype-phenotype correlations have been discovered in the course of observational studies performed during randomized clinical trials. For example, a randomized clinical trial was performed to compare the efficacy of different formulations of interferon alpha in the treatment of chronic infection with hepatitis C. A subsequent observational study used a GWAS to identify variation near the IL28B gene as strongly correlated with response to treatment (Ge et al. 2009). Tests for the genetic variants identified in this study are already in widespread clinical use (PRNewswire 2011; Scripps Health 2011).

The enrollment of individuals in these studies had no bearing on their diagnoses, treatments, or in most cases, anything else in their lives. The goal of these observational studies was simply to ask the question "Are there gene variants in the general population that are associated with who ends up with a particular diagnosis or experiences a particular treatment response?"

While observational studies will be primary tools used to develop hypotheses about new and clinically useful ways to group patients, the findings emerging from such studies will need confirmation and investigation using other approaches. For example, there are likely to be a great many ways to classify patients based on molecular data, and only some will have clinical utility. In general, clinical utility will need to be evaluated using randomized clinical trials.

Observational studies will also need to be followed by functional studies that seek to determine the mechanistic basis of observed molecular associations with clinical outcomes. An example of this type of combined discovery path is the identification of BCL11 as a modifier of the severity of sickle cell disease. Initially implicated in this role in GWAS studies, the biological basis of the association was quickly determined by focused analyses that established that BCL11A acts as a repressor of fetal hemoglobin. It is the persistence of fetal hemoglobin into adulthood in patients with particular variants at the BCL11 locus that ameliorates the symptoms of sickle cell disease (Sankaran et al. 2008). We anticipate that laboratory-based research of this sort will be essential to elucidate the underlying reasons for observed associations between molecular data and clinical outcomes and that these mechanistic insights will play an essential part in establishing the Knowledge Network and guiding its use.

The Committee envisions pilot studies that would:

1. Be of a sufficient size, as well as scientific and organizational complexity, to reveal on the basis of actual experience the most significant barriers to the development of point-of-care discovery efforts.
2. Address one or more unmet medical needs for which deeper biological understanding of a disorder would likely lead to near-term changes in treatment paradigms and health outcomes.
3. Include the generation and analysis of a range of molecular-data types potentially including, but not limited to genomic data (sequence and expression), metabolomic data, proteomic data, and/or microbiome data.
4. Be led by an organization charged with delivering health care with strong partnerships with researchers.
5. Be supported by research funding to establish a "proof of principle."
6. Involve partnerships with a broad array of stakeholders, both public and private, including health-care providers, patients, payers, and scientists with expertise in genomics, epidemiology, social science, and molecular biology.
7. Seek to remove barriers to data sharing and provide an ethical and legal framework for protecting and respecting individual rights.

8. Develop IT networks of sufficient scale to allow assembly analysis and sharing of the integrated datasets.
9. Draw on laboratory research to assess the biological underpinnings of associations between molecular data and clinical outcomes.
10. Establish validation standards for clinical, evidence-based decision-making.

Below, we outline two example pilot studies; the first, "The Million American Genomes Initiative", is selected to pilot the use of one of the key layers of 'omic information that is "ready to go". This pilot project would help to populate the Information Commons with relevant data and facilitate learning how to establish connections with other layers. By focusing on health care recipients in diverse states of health and disease, this project would also help evaluate the new discovery paradigm by allowing correlations to be made between germline sequences and a vast range of phenotypes. The second "Metabolomic Profiles in Type 2 Diabetes" is disease specific and is designed to ensure the early introduction of a different 'omic layer (metabolomics) into the Information Commons and to pilot evaluation of more targeted questions in the new discovery paradigm.

EXAMPLE PILOT STUDY 1:
THE MILLION AMERICAN GENOMES INITIATIVE (MAGI)

A natural pilot study that would contribute to the development of the Information Commons and Knowledge Network of Disease would involve the sequencing of the genomes of one million or more individuals and the establishment of appropriate infrastructure for drawing correlations between the sequence data and the medical histories of these individuals. In focusing on a pilot study involving complete sequence data, we do not intend to elevate sequence data above other data in their importance to the Knowledge Network. Instead, this proposal recognizes that sequencing methods are "ready to go," or nearly so, for very-large-scale implementation and the acquisition of such data in a point-of-care setting would, of necessity, require addressing key challenges related to informed consent, protection of data, data storage, and data analysis that will be common to all types of data. This proposal also recognizes that sequencing on this scale will inevitably be undertaken in the near future in an effort to make connections between human-genome-sequence data and common diseases. We view it as important to the development of the Knowledge Network that this effort be grounded in the new discovery model, which would make possible systematic comparisons of the molecular data with electronic medical records, now and into the future: that is, the study design should allow correlations between genotypes determined now and health outcomes that occur years or decades later.

The sequencing of one million genomes would include a sufficient range of individuals with different health outcomes and sufficient statistical power to detect associations. For example, amoxicillin-clavulanic acid is a widely used antibiotic that causes severe liver injury in one out of approximately 15,000 exposures. In a one-million-patient sample we would expect to include many individuals with this—and other similarly rare—adverse drug reactions and other medical conditions. It is also essential that the sample size be large enough to build a concrete picture of the distribution of gene variants in individuals free of specific diagnoses.

EXAMPLE PILOT STUDY 2:
METABOLOMIC PROFILES IN TYPE 2 DIABETES

Recent metabolomic profiling of blood samples from individuals who subsequently developed type 2 diabetes showed marked differences in the characteristics of branched-chain amino acids sampled from blood draws (Wang et al. 2011). These early analyses suggest the potential of metabolomic analyses to help identify those individuals at most risk of developing diabetes, and in particular, may help to elucidate the physiological steps involved in the transition between insulin-resistant pre-diabetes and full-blown diabetes. We therefore envision a pilot project focused on understanding this transition using metabolomic profiles in blood. This work would begin with targeted quantitative metabolomic studies transitioning toward more comprehensive metabolomic profiles over time. Such an effort, combined with knowledge gained from Pilot 1 and research from other layers of the Information Commons (such as the microbiome and exposome) could contribute substantially to strategies to delay or prevent the development of type 2 diabetes.

ANTICIPATED OUTCOMES OF THE PILOT STUDIES

The pilot studies are intended to lead to new connections between genetic or metabolomic variation and disease subclassifications, often with implications for disease management and prevention. More importantly, they will provide the lessons necessary to facilitate a more rapid transition in the way molecular data are used. For example, pilot projects of sufficient scope and scale could lead to the development of new discovery models, including those in which patient groups self-organize in recognition of shared clinical features and then pursue efforts to generate relevant molecular data. Such an initiative also would permit many logistical, ethical, and bioinformatic challenges to be addressed in ways that would benefit future efforts and lead toward the sustainable implementation of point-of-care discovery efforts.

A RESEARCH MODEL BASED ON OPEN DATA
SHARING REQUIRES CHANGES TO DATA ACCESS,
CONSENT, AND SHARING POLICIES

Research to develop a Knowledge Network of Disease will need to resolve complex ethical and policy challenges including consent, confidentiality, return of individual results to patients, and oversight (Cambon-Thomsen et al. 2007; Greely 2007; Hall et al. 2010).

The Committee's vision of a Knowledge Network of Disease and its associated benefits for future patients will become a reality only if the public supports a new balance between research access to materials and clinical data and respect for the values and preferences of donors. Ultimately, there should be no dichotomy between "patient data or materials" and "those who benefit from this research." The patients who are giving their materials and data for research would also receive the benefits of research leading to a Knowledge Network and the resulting new molecularly-based taxonomy.

How might these ethical and policy challenges be resolved so that the pilot studies described previously might be carried out? The Committee recommends that an appropriate federal agency initiate a process to assess the privacy issues associated with the research required to create the Knowledge Network and Information Commons. Because these issues have been studied extensively, this process need not start from scratch. However, in practical terms, investigators who wish to participate in the pilot studies discussed above—and the Institutional Review Boards who must approve their human-subjects protocols—will need specific guidance on the range of informed-consent processes appropriate for these projects. Subject to the constraints of current law and prevailing ethical standards, the Committee encourages as much flexibility as possible in the guidance provided. As much as possible, on-the-ground experience in pilot projects carried out in diverse health-care settings, rather than top-down dictates, should govern the emergence of best practices in this sensitive area, whose handling will have a make-or-break influence on the entire Information Commons/Knowledge Network/New Taxonomy initiative. Inclusion of health-care providers and other stakeholders outside the academic community will be essential.

An approach to these issues might include:

1. *Intensive dialog about the benefits of an Information Commons containing individual-centric data about health and disease. This dialog should include researchers and the public, patient representatives, and disease advocacy groups.* Reaching out to communities that have been suspicious of research because of historical abuses would strengthen trust. At the workshop the Committee convened, we heard patient advocates and public representatives argue forcefully that more trans-

parency regarding research and more collaboration among researchers, research institutions, and the public would facilitate research. For example, when constructively engaged, advocacy groups have advanced biomedical research by helping to design studies that are attractive to patients, publicized the projects, helped to recruit participants, and raised money to help pay for the research (Giusti 2011; Patients LikeMe.com 2011).

2. *Exploration of approaches to informed consent that would allow patients to give broad consent for future studies whose details remain unspecified.* Once provided with concise, understandable information on how their data and biological materials would be used for research, many patients are willing to consent provided they are treated as true partners in an activity that will provide broad public benefit (IOM 2010a; Trinidad et al. 2011). On the other hand, some patients will object generally to the research use of "leftover" specimens originally collected for clinical purposes or, more narrowly, object to their use in certain types of research. These concerns must be carefully addressed. Current approaches to informed consent for research rely on long, complex consent forms that may deter participation while doing little to help participants understand the nature of the research. As noted below, the Health Insurance Portability and Accountability Act (HIPAA) requires authorization or waiver for each specific research study: common interpretations of this requirement are so restrictive that investigators and Institutional Review Boards thwart or substantially delay research of the type that will be needed to develop the Information Commons.

3. *Strong public representation and input on oversight and governance.* Public participation in biobanks and research projects would build trust (Levy et al. 2010) and help resolve issues that arise in the course of research, such as whether to offer to return individual research results to persons whose biological materials are analyzed (Beskow et al. 2010a) As noted earlier, the gray areas around the potential that researchers may have a "duty to inform" participants of clinically relevant results need to be clarified.

The HIPAA required the federal government to develop regulations for protecting the privacy of personal health information. The HIPAA privacy regulations, which are intended to protect patient privacy, inhibit research that requires widespread sharing and multi-purpose use of data on individual patients in several ways (IOM 2009): First, rich molecular data about an individual (particularly whole-genome sequencing) could be considered a unique biological identifier under HIPAA, even if overt identifiers are removed. Although a waiver of authorization to use identifiable health information may be granted under certain circumstances, many health-care organizations are reluctant to participate. Secondly, because HIPAA does not allow authorization for unspecified future research or for several projects at one time, authorization must be given for each specific use of patient data. Thirdly, requirements for "accounting" to patients for research uses of data are burdensome and discourage data sharing. These regulations are strong deterrents to the kinds of pilot projects envisaged in this report.

The Committee found a need to re-interpret—or perhaps reformulate— HIPAA regulations, and is in agreement with the 2009 IOM report "Beyond the HIPAA Privacy Rule: Enhancing Privacy, Improving Health Through Research," which found that the HIPAA privacy rule fails to protect privacy as intended (IOM 2009), and, as currently implemented, impedes important health research and imposes burdensome administrative requirements (IOM 2009). This IOM report concluded that stricter security would be a better approach to protect privacy than requiring patient authorization to use identifiable data for research. It recommended that much research based on existing materials and data be exempted from an amended HIPAA privacy rule (IOM 2009). For example, the Committee suggested that researchers be allowed to work with "secure, trusted, non-conflicted intermediaries that could develop a protocol, or key," for linking identifiable data from different sources (IOM 2009). A biobank might serve as a trusted intermediary for the pilot projects described above, giving researchers only data and materials without overt identifiers but retaining a key to coded samples so they could update clinical information or re-contact patients or donors when appropriate. Furthermore, the IOM report recommended that "researchers, institutions, and organizations that store personally identifiable data should establish strong security safeguards and set limits on access to data" (IOM 2009). These precautions might include, for example, requirements for physical security of data and provisions in materials and data-transfer agreements that forbid researchers who receive de-identified data from trying to re-identify patients or donors or to contact them directly.

Furthermore, new approaches to informed consent are being proposed and tested. Some examples include: (1) incorporating highly specific patient preferences regarding use of their personal health information data (PCAST 2010), (2) using a short form for informed consent for participating in biobanks, with additional supplemental information for participants who desire more information (Beskow et al. 2010b), (3) de-identified data-based, opt-out model used by Vanderbilt and i2b2 (Pulley et al. 2010), and (4) consent for whole genome sequencing and study of all phenotypes, coupled with respect for individualized preferences regarding the return of clinically validated results (Biesecker et al. 2009). The Committee envisages that best practices and ultimately consensus standards will emerge from the different models of consent and return of clinically significant results to participants.

PRECOMPETITIVE COLLABORATIONS

To accelerate the development of new tests and products based on a Knowledge Network of Disease, precompetitive collaboration between nonprofits and industry and among different for-profit companies would be desirable (IOM 2010b, 2011). The research needed to build the Information Commons, which will require projects involving vast amounts of data from large numbers of patients, will proceed more efficiently if such collaborations can be developed both between academia and industry and among for-profit companies that have historically been competitors (Altshuler et al. 2010).

These collaborations could include developing common standards and database formats and building infrastructure to facilitate data sharing. Consortia might be organized to share upstream research findings widely that have no immediate market potential but are critical to downstream product development. Examples of such upstream research include the identification and validation of biomarkers and predictors of adverse drug reactions. To build a flourishing culture of precompetitive collaboration, drug companies will need to overcome their reluctance to share all data from completed clinical trials, not just the selected data relevant to regulatory proceedings. Finally, and most significantly, guidelines for intellectual property need to be clarified and concerns about loss of intellectual-property rights addressed. Precompetitive collaborations will only emerge if individuals and organizations have incentives to join them (Vargas et al. 2010). The Committee believes that without such incentives, it will prove difficult or impossible to collect the new information that must be acquired before precision medicine, with its attendant benefits in improved health outcomes and reduced health-care costs, can become a widespread reality.

Similar principles apply whether the collaborations involve commercial entities or are confined to academia. To encourage the collection of materials and data, organizations and researchers who collect them should have first access to their use for research, while still ensuring their timely availability to others. The Committee does not envision the desirability or need, in the context of the research required to populate the Information Commons with data and derive a Knowledge Network from it, for the instant-data-release model adopted during the Human Genome Project. However, it does believe that timely, unrestricted access to datasets by researchers with no connections to the investigators who created them will be essential. The cost of populating the Information Commons with data precludes extensive redundancy in publicly financed research projects. At the same time, the size and complexity of these datasets—as well as the need for diverse, competitive inputs to their analysis—precludes giving any one group prolonged control over them. They must be regarded as public resources available for widespread and diverse research into ways to improve health care and to increase the efficiency of health care delivery.

Because the Committee is skeptical that one-size-fits-all policies can accommodate the conflicting values associated with incentivizing researchers and insuring adequate access to data, it believes that pilot projects of increasing scope and scale should put substantial emphasis on addressing the challenges associated with data sharing, rather than focusing exclusively on data collection and analysis.

COMPETITION AND SHARING IN THE HEALTH-CARE SYSTEM

A distinct and critical question is whether payers, such as health insurance companies, will provide access to their vast databases of patient and outcomes data and whether they will be willing to integrate these data with data from other companies and researchers with the goal of creating Knowledge Networks such as those described in Chapter 3. On one hand, these organizations recognize the potential value and cost saving that could emerge from such an effort. On the other hand there are considerable impediments. One of the main impediments is cultural: many of these organizations view their data as a propriety asset to be used in efforts to generate competitive advantages relative to other organizations. For example, large health-care systems and insurance providers are interested in developing decision-support tools for physicians that would cut down on the substantial waste caused by misdiagnosis or inappropriate treatment decisions. Integration of biological data, patient data, and outcomes information into Knowledge Networks that aggregate data from many sources could dramatically accelerate such efforts. However, if the data and the research results are shared, it would undermine one type of competitive advantage that large data providers might otherwise have. In this way, there is a tension between the sharing that would be good for the health-care system as a whole and the short-term competitive instincts of individual providers and payers.

Apart from the culture of competition there are other impediments related to cost pressures. Cost pressures within the health-care system are such that providers and payers are unlikely to be willing to invest substantially (or in some cases, at all) in the collection of biological data for research purposes. Over the long term, once such data have been shown to yield clinically useful information, it will become justifiable to expend health-care resources on the collection of actionable data, just as is presently done for standard diagnostic tests. However, until such data are shown to be clinically useful, it is unrealistic to expect that the Information Commons will become populated by biological data (such as genome sequences) acquired from providers and payers. Similarly, the information technology challenges associated with integration of large datasets and new disease classification systems are substantial. For example, Aetna is currently engaged in a multi-year effort to update its information technology systems to support the planned conversion to the ICD-10 coding standards. This effort alone will cost tens of millions of dollars. While the goals of integrating datasets and changing classification systems are achievable in principle, they will be beyond the technical capacity of all but the largest and most technologically sophisticated providers and payers. Thus, the transition to non-proprietary Knowledge Networks into which all data would be deposited would have to involve strong incentives for payers and providers. This may mean that the government will ultimately need to require participation in such Knowledge Networks for reimbursement of health care expenses. At an even more fundamental level, the longstanding issue of equity in access to a sufficiently advanced level of health care should also be addressed if the data in the Knowledge Network is to adequately represent the diversity of our society.

THE DEVELOPMENT OF A KNOWLEDGE NETWORK OF DISEASE WILL REQUIRE AND INFORM THE EDUCATION OF HEALTH-CARE PROVIDERS AT ALL LEVELS

Decision-making based on a Knowledge Network of Disease and the New Taxonomy, which will incorporate a multitude of parameters, will represent a significant adjustment in the practical work of the primary care physician. Given the demands on the time of physicians and other care-givers in the present health-care environment, few are likely to have the time or to feel qualified to interpret the results of "omics"-scale analyses of their patients. The importance of this issue will escalate over time as the Knowledge Network and its linked molecular-based taxonomy evolve into a system whose sheer complexity greatly exceeds current approaches to disease classification.

One concern is that the infusion of large molecular datasets into clinical records will reinforce a tendency many perceive as already crediting genetic and other molecular findings with more weight than they deserve. In extreme cases, this cultural bias has enabled the promoting and marketing of "omic" tests with no clinical value whatsoever (Kolata 2011). In other cases genetic or "omic" tests with real value in specific contexts may be over-interpreted and thereby occlude consideration of other relevant clinical data. To develop the Knowledge Network of Disease and the New Taxonomy that will be derived from it, health-care providers will need to develop much greater literacy in the interpretation and application of molecular data.

To meet these challenges, health-care providers will require both decision-support systems and new training paradigms. The decision-support systems will need to provide useful information about the propensity of patients to develop disease, facilitate a correct diagnosis, guide selection of the most appropriate strategies for disease prevention or treatment, inform the patient about the prognosis and management of the disease, and provide the opportunity for both physicians and patients to access more detailed information about the disease on an "as interested" or "as needed" basis. Whenever possible, such decision-support systems should enable shared decision-making by patients and

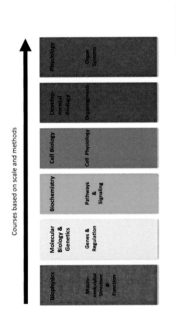

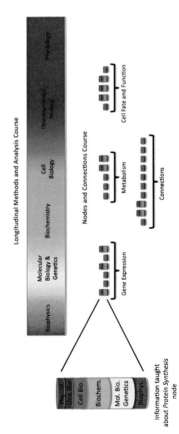

FIGURE 4-1 Curriculum for biomedical graduate program—proposed new model.
The current model of the first-year curriculum in a typical biomedical graduate program (top) and an alternative model (bottom). The multicolored bars in the nodes and connections course represent fundamental principles and essential facts about each key process integrated across scales.
SOURCE: Modified with permission from Lorsch 2011.

their care-givers. Such systems should be readily updatable as more information is acquired about disease classification, the ability of particular test results to predict disease development, progression, or response to treatment, and the success of particular disease-prevention and management strategies.

In order to prepare physicians for the use of a comprehensive, dynamically changing Knowledge Network, biomedical education will need to adjust. Lorsch and Nichols (2011) recently proposed that graduate and medical life sciences curricula would significantly benefit from a major shift away from the current discipline-specific model to a vertically integrated nodes-and-connections framework (see Figure 4-1). This model is not the only possible way of reorganizing instruction to reflect new knowledge about molecular processes, but it demonstrates how the development of a molecularly-based taxonomy, and the underlying Knowledge Network of Disease, could lead to major changes in education, while preparing students pursuing research careers to function in a scientific landscape that increasingly requires multidisciplinary approaches to solve biomedical problems (NRC 2009; MIT 2011). It also would give future physicians a more holistic view of biological processes, which reflects what will be required to fulfill the promises of genomics and personalized medicine (Ashley et al. 2010; Wiener et al. 2010).

The teaching model proposed by Lorsch and Nichols very closely mirrors the properties of the Knowledge Network of Disease described in Chapter 3. In this teaching model a given topic—for example, gene expression—would be taught in a vertically integrated fashion, with essential information all the way from the atomic to the whole-organism scale discussed. Adjusting teaching strategies to reflect the biological reality of the material has the potential to create significant synergies. Students may retain more knowledge of basic science when this information is directly connected to medicine. The enhanced ability to use the New Taxonomy in medical practice and research would reinforce the student's conception of biology. Although it is beyond the scope of this report to suggest detailed reforms of the medical-school curriculum, the Committee would like to emphasize that full realization of the power of the Knowledge Network of Disease and the New Taxonomy derived from it would almost certainly require a major shift in educational strategy.

5

Epilogue

Chapter 1 opened with two illustrative clinical scenarios. Although not based on specific patients, these scenarios reflect current medical practice and are typical of thousands of real people who visit American clinics every day.[1] Patient 1—an otherwise healthy woman with breast cancer—is a direct beneficiary of the stunning advances in science and medicine that have occurred during recent decades. Her physician knows the molecular details of the pathological processes that threaten her life and has at her command therapies that directly target the aberrant molecular events occurring in Patient 1's cells. The safety and efficacy of these therapies have been confirmed by randomized clinical trials involving other patients well matched with Patient 1 in the molecular details of their disease. Her prognosis is excellent. With continuing advances in science and medicine, similar patients with this type of breast cancer, whose molecular pathology we are beginning to understand, may expect access to treatments that are even safer, more effective, less expensive, and have fewer side effects.

Patient 2 presents a different story. Contemporary medicine has little to offer him beyond a long-available diagnosis and treatment plan. After 50 years of intensive study, substantial headway has been made in the scientific understanding of diabetes. Unlike many children who have a sudden onset of diabetes early in life, we know that Patient 2 has high levels of circulating insulin. His physician may ultimately consider attempting to control his diabetes with still more insulin, but the fundamental problem in this case—and with millions of

---

[1] In 2010, approximately 1.9 million men and women were diagnosed with diabetes, and approximately 261,100 individuals were diagnosed with breast cancer in the United States. [Source: http://www.diabetes.org/diabetes-basics/diabetes-statistics/ and http://www.breastcancer.org/symptoms/understand_bc/statistics.jsp?gclid=CLeJwq7p76sCFUld5QodLz1TLw, http://www.cancer.org/Cancer/BreastCancer/OverviewGuide/breast-cancer-overview-key-statistics.]

other patients with type 2 diabetes—is that his cells respond only weakly to insulin. His blood sugar remains abnormally high even as his cells receive a strong signal to take the sugar up and metabolize it. The insidiously toxic effects of high levels of circulating sugar threaten the health of Patient 2's blood vessels. As they age, many type 2 diabetics suffer severe consequences of a deteriorating vasculature. When minor wounds to their feet fail to heal, they often face amputation. As capillaries in their retinas rupture, many go blind. Responses to drug treatments, which have changed little for decades, are highly variable. Similarly, changes in exercise habits and diet help some patients more than others. There is a high likelihood that Patient 2 faces a future of escalating medical interventions, declining health, and increasing disability. The human, social, and economic costs associated with patients such as Patient 2 are daunting and distressingly typical of those seen for patients with chronic diseases throughout our aging population.

The Committee's assigned task was to "explore the feasibility and need, and develop a potential framework, for creating a 'New Taxonomy' of human diseases based on molecular biology." While the adjective "new" in the Committee's charge provoked much lively discussion—there were varying opinions as to whether a new disease classification would be likely to differ dramatically in kind from existing taxonomies—there was immediate consensus on the more important point: everyone on the Committee agreed that a *better* taxonomy is needed and that we have a spectacular opportunity to create one. Moreover, the Committee clearly recognized that developing and implementing a Knowledge Network of Disease has the unique potential to go far beyond classification of disease to act as a catalyst that would help to revolutionize the way research is done and patients are treated. Patient 1 has a high likelihood of overcoming her life-threatening disease and going on to live a long, healthy, and productive life. These prospects are a direct result of a new ability to recognize, based on molecular analyses, the precise type of breast cancer she has and to target a rational therapy to her disease. The Committee believes that the best prospects for creating a similarly bright future for Patient 2 lies in achieving a similarly precise understanding of his disease by creating a Knowledge Network of Disease and an associated New Taxonomy.

The Committee recognized two key points about its charge: first, development of an improved disease taxonomy is only one facet, albeit an important one, of the challenge of leveraging advances in biomedical research to achieve better health outcomes for patients; secondly, no single stream of activity—led by any single segment of the biomedical research community—can tackle even this limited goal on its own. Both these points suggested that we could best address our charge by framing the "new-taxonomy" challenge broadly. Many of the conclusions and recommendations could apply, as well, to other challenges in "translational research" such as evaluating and refining existing treatments and developing new ones. However, disease classification is inextricably linked to all progress in medicine, and the Committee took the view that an ambitious initiative to address this challenge—and particularly to modernize the "discovery model" for the needed research—is an excellent place to start. The Committee thinks that the key to success lies in building new relationships that must span the whole spectrum of research and patient-care activities that comprise American medicine. As discussed in Chapter 2, the Committee thinks that now is a propitious time to confront the challenge of developing a Knowledge Network of Disease and deriving a New Taxonomy from it because of changes that are sweeping across basic and translational research, information technology, drug development, public attitudes, and the health-care-delivery system.

Our recommendations seek to empower stakeholder communities by providing them with informational resources—the Information Commons, the Knowledge Network, and the New Taxonomy itself—that would transform the way they work and make decisions. We make no specific promises about the benefits that would ensue as this transformation occurs but have every confidence that this initiative would be a powerful, constructive force for change throughout a large enterprise that plays an increasingly central role in science, technology, the economy, and each of our lives—and one that is notoriously difficult to reform.

At the core of the Committee's optimism is a conviction that dramatic advances in biological knowledge can be coupled more effectively than they are now to the goal of improving the health outcomes of individual patients. Biology has flourished in the 50+ years since the discovery of the molecular basis of inheritance. Powerfully reinforced by the Human Genome Project, genetics is in a "golden age" of discovery. Sequence similarity between genes studied in fruit flies and those studied in humans allows nearly instant recognition of the potential medical relevance of the most basic advances in biochemistry and cell biology. Increasingly, this process also works in reverse: unusual human patients call attention to molecules and biochemical pathways whose importance in basic biology had been overlooked or was otherwise inaccessible. Indeed, there are already many areas of basic biology in which human studies are leading the way to deep new insights into the way organisms work. A good example is color vision. For the simple reason that one can ask a research subject what she sees when looking at a pattern of light—instead of having to develop a crude behavioral test to find out whether she sees anything at all—we know far more about the molecular details of light reception in humans than we could ever have learned from studying mice. Particularly as biomcdical research puts an increasing emphasis on unraveling the molecular underpinnings of behavior, the advantages of starting research studies with humans, rather than model organisms, are likely to grow. Experience tells us that translation of intensifying knowledge of basic biology into clinical advances is a daunting task. Nonetheless, the many examples of success encourage optimism. Furthermore, the Committee shares the sense that basic biology is at an "inflection point" in

which there is every reason to expect increasing payoffs from the large investments in basic science that have brought us to this point. However, the grand
challenge of coupling basic science more effectively to medicine will require
a rethinking of current practices on a scale commensurate with the challenge.
The Committee regards the initiative it proposes to develop the tripartite Information Commons, Knowledge Network, and New Taxonomy, as having the
potential to rise to this level.

Information technology is the key contributor to the technological convergence the Committee perceives. Information technology, quite simply, has made
the rise of data-intensive biology possible: molecular biology, as now practiced,
could not exist without modern computing systems. In medicine, information
technology offers perhaps the best hope of increasing efficiency and improving our collective learning about what works and what does not. Throughout
society, technology is changing attitudes toward information. In a mere 20
years, people have made the transition from regarding most human knowledge
as locked away in the dusty backrooms of research libraries to expecting it to
be at their finger tips. Understandably, the public is losing patience with barriers to the sharing and dissemination of information. The social-networking
phenomenon is a particularly dramatic illustration of changing attitudes toward
information and associated blurring of the line between the public and private.
For all these reasons, the Committee sees powerful forces converging in a way
that favors the dismantling of existing barriers—institutional, cultural, economic, and legal—between the biomedical research environment, the clinic,
and the public.

The Committee recognizes that some aspects of the world we envision are
more readily approachable than others. Even the easiest steps will be challeng-
ing. As emphasized throughout this report, there are many impediments to
progress along the path we outline. That is the reason the Committee recommends pilot projects of increasing scope and scale as the vehicle for moving
forward. Although we consider the creation of an improved classification of
disease valuable in its own right, we do not recommend a crash program to
pursue this goal in isolation from the broader reforms we emphasize. We regard
smaller projects on the recommended path as preferable to larger, narrower
initiatives that would distract attention and resources from these reforms. We
think the impediments can best be overcome and the optimum design of the
Information Commons, Knowledge Network, and the New Taxonomy best
emerge in the context of pilot projects of increasing scope and scale.

Even some stakeholders in the health-care system who find the Committee's basic vision compelling may ask whether or not a special, organized effort
is required to achieve the Committee's goals. In particular, some might argue
that there are already enough examples—many have been cited in this report—
in which data-intensive laboratory tests have such clear benefits for patients
that the traditional system of test development and insurance reimbursement

will allow a smooth transition to a new era of molecular medicine. We would caution against this conclusion. Indeed, there is real risk of a backlash against premature claims of the efficacy of genomic medicine (Kolata 2011). The key to avoiding such a backlash is development of a robust system for discovering applications that have real clinical benefits and validating those claims through open processes. The Committee believes that expecting or pressuring payers in the health-care system to bear the costs of integrating data-intensive biology and medicine without clear evidence of the safety, efficacy, and economic feasibility of particular applications would fail—indeed, such an effort could easily be counter-productive. On the other hand, as some of the scenarios sketched above indicate, the Committee believes that a well planned public investment in creating the system the Committee envisions would lead relatively quickly to robust public–private partnerships that would allow all stakeholders to build on early successes. Perhaps even more importantly, the Committee believes that its approach offers the most realistic available path to ultimate sustainability of precision medicine. Public investment in research can play an essential role in building a solid foundation for precision medicine, but it cannot sustain its dissemination: precision medicine will only become a routine aspect of health care when it pays its own way.

To bring the discussion back to the Committee's core mission, we close by re-emphasizing our view toward disease taxonomy. Diagnosis is the foundation of medicine. Accurately and precisely defining a patient's condition does not assure effective treatment, but it is unequivocally the place to start. Hence, in exploiting the convergent forces acting throughout the health-care system, a long-term focus on developing the new informational resources proposed in this report would be a powerful unifying principle for biomedical researchers, physicians, patients, and all stakeholders in this vast enterprise. Whether the payoff from such a commitment would occur in time to help Patient 2, the 40-year-old type II diabetic described at the beginning of this report, is impossible to say. However, the Committee believes that implementation of its core recommendations would bring many new allies to the cause of improving this patient's health prospects and would equip these diverse players with powerful new tools and resources that are unlikely to emerge without an organized effort to create them.

References

ACS (American Cancer Society). 2011. Cancer Facts & Figure 2011. American Cancer Society [online]. Available: http://www.cancer.org/acs/groups/content/@epidemiologysurveilance/documents/document/acspc-029771.pdf [accessed August 18, 2011].

A.D.A.M. Medical Encyclopedia. 2011. Type 2 diabetes. PubMedHealth [online]. Available: http://www.ncbi.nlm.nih.gov/pubmedhealth/PMH0001356/ [accessed October 4, 2011].

Alexeeff, S.E., B.A. Coull, A. Gryparis, H. Suh, D. Sparrow, P.S. Vokonas, and J. Schwartz. 2011. Medium-term exposure to traffic-related air pollution and markers of inflammation and endothelial function. Environ. Health Perspect. 119(4):481-486.

Alizadeh, A.A., M.B. Eisen, R.E. Davis, C. Ma, I.S. Lossos, A. Rosenwald, J.C. Boldrick, H. Sabet, T. Tran, X. Yu, J.I. Powell, L. Yang, G.E. Marti, T. Moore, J. Hudson, Jr., L. Lu, D.B. Lewis, R. Tibshirani, G. Sherlock, W.C. Chan, T.C. Greiner, D.D. Weisenburger, J.O. Armitage, R. Warnke, R. Levy, W. Wilson, M.R. Grever, J.C. Byrd, D. Botstein, P.O. Brown, and L.M. Staudt. 2000. Distinct types of diffuse large B-cell lymphoma identified by gene expression profiling. Nature 403(6769):503-511.

Altshuler, J.S., E. Balogh, A.D. Barker, S.L. Eck, S.H. Friend, G.S. Ginsburg, R.S. Herbst, S.J. Nass, C.M. Streeter, and J.A. Wagner. 2010. Opening up to precompetitive collaboration. Sci. Transl. Med. 2(52):52cm26.

Anderson, K.M., P.W. Wilson, P.M. Odell, and W.B. Kannel. 1991. An updated coronary risk profile. A statement for health professionals. Circulation 83(1):356-362.

Andrews, L.B., and A.S. Jaeger. 1991. Confidentiality of genetic information in the workplace. Am. J. Law Med. 17(1-2):75-108.

Arem, H., M.L. Irwin, Y. Zhou, L. Lu, H. Risch, and H. Yu. 2011. Physical activity and endometrial cancer in a population-based case-control study. Cancer Causes Control 22(2):219-226.

Arrowsmith, J. 2011a. Trial watch: Phase II failures: 2008-2010. Nat. Rev. Drug Discov. 10(5):328-329.

Arrowsmith, J. 2011b. Trial watch: Phase III and submission failures: 2007-2010. Nat. Rev. Drug Discov. 10(2):87.

Ashley, E.A., A.J. Butte, M.T. Wheeler, R. Chen, T.E. Klein, F.E. Dewey, J.T. Dudley, K.E. Ormond, A. Pavlovic, A.A. Morgan, D. Pushkarev, N.F. Neff, L. Hudgins, L. Gong, L.M. Hodges, D.S. Berlin, C.F. Thorn, K. Sangkuhl, J.M. Hebert, M. Woon, H. Sagreiya, R. Whaley, J.W. Knowles, M.F. Chou, J.V. Thakuria, A.M. Rosenbaum, A.W. Zaranek, G.M. Church, H.T. Greely, S.R. Quake, and R.B. Altman. 2010. Clinical assessment incorporating a personal genome. Lancet 375(9725):1525-1535.

Atherton, J.C. 2006. The pathogenesis of *Helicobacter pylori*-induced gastro-duodenal diseases. Annu. Rev. Pathol. 1:63-96.

Benson, D.A., I. Karsch-Mizrachi, D.J. Lipman, J. Ostell, and E.W. Sayers. 2011. GenBank. Nucleic Acids Res. 39:D32-37.

Beskow, L.M., K.N. Linney, R.A. Radtke, E.L. Heinzen, and D.B. Goldstein. 2010a. Ethical challenges in genotype-driven research recruitment. Genome Res. 20(6):705-709.

Beskow, L.M., J.Y. Friedman, N.C. Hardy, L. Lin, and K.P. Weinfurt. 2010b. Developing a simplified consent form for biobanking. PLoS One 5(10):e13302.

Biesecker, L.G., J.C. Mullikin, F.M. Facio, C. Turner, P.F. Cherukuri, R.W. Blakesley, G.G. Bouffard, P.S. Chines, P. Cruz, N.F. Hansen, J.K. Teer, B. Maskeri, A.C. Young, T.A. Manolio, A.F. Wilson, T. Finkel, P. Hwang, A. Arai, A.T. Remaley, V. Sachdev, R. Shamburek, R.O. Cannon, and E.D. Green. 2009. The ClinSeq project: Piloting large-scale genome sequencing for research in genomic medicine. Genome Res. 19(9):1665-1674.

Blaser, M.J., and S. Falkow. 2009. What are the consequences of the disappearing human microbiota? Nat. Rev. Microbiol. 7(12):887-894.

Boehme, C.C., P. Nabeta, D. Hillemann, M.P. Nicol, S. Shenai, F. Krapp, J. Allen, R. Tahirli, R. Blakemore, R. Rustomjee, A. Milovic, M. Jones, S.M. O'Brien, D.H. Persing, S. Ruesch-Gerdes, E. Gotuzzo, C. Rodrigues, D. Alland, and M.D. Perkins. 2010. Rapid molecular detection of tuberculosis and rifampin resistance. N. Engl. J. Med. 363(11):1005-1015.

Brookhart, M.A., B.D. Bradbury, J. Avorn, S. Schneeweiss, and W.C. Winkelmayer. 2011. The effect of altitude change on anemia treatment response in hemodialysis patients. Am. J. Epidemiol. 173(7):768-777.

Brownstein, J.S., C.C. Freifeld, B.Y. Reis, and K.D. Mandl. 2008. Surveillance Sans Frontières: Internet-based emerging infectious disease intelligence and the HealthMap project. PLoS Med. 5(7):e151.

Brownstein, J.S., C.C. Freifeld, and L.C. Madoff. 2009. Digital disease detection: Harnessing the Web for public health surveillance. N. Engl. J. Med. 360(21):2153-2155.

Brownstein, J.S., S.N. Murphy, A.B. Goldfine, R.W. Grant, M. Sordo, V. Gainer, J.A. Colecchi, A. Dubey, D.M. Nathan, J.P. Glaser, and I.S. Kohane. 2010a. Rapid identification of myocardial infarction risk associated with diabetes medications using electronic medical records. Diabetes Care 33(3):526-531.

Brownstein, J.S., C.C. Freifeld, E.H. Chan, M. Keller, A.L. Sonricker, S.R. Mekaru, and L. Buckeridge. 2010b. Information technology and global surveillance of cases of 2009 H1N1 influenza. N. Engl. J. Med. 362(18):1731-1735.

Bruce, M.A., B.M. Beech, M. Sims, T.N. Brown, S.B. Wyatt, H.A. Taylor, D.R. Williams, and E. Crook. 2009. Social environmental stressors, psychological factors, and kidney disease. J. Investig. Med. 57(4):583-589.

Cambon-Thomsen, A., E. Rial-Sebbag, and B.M. Knoppers. 2007. Trends in ethical and legal frameworks for the use of human biobanks. Eur. Respir. J. 30(2):373-382.

Campa, D., R. Kaaks, L. Le Marchand, C.A. Haiman, R.C. Travis, C.D. Berg, J.E. Buring, S.J. Chanock, W.R. Diver, L. Dostal, A. Fournier, S.E. Hankinson, B.E. Henderson, R.N. Hoover, C. Isaacs, M. Johansson, L.N. Kolonel, P. Kraft, I.M. Lee, C.A. McCarty, K. Overvad, S. Panico, P.H. Peeters, E. Riboli, M.J. Sanchez, F.R. Schumacher, G. Skeie, D.O. Stram, M.J. Thun, D. Trichopoulos, S. Zhang, R.G. Ziegler, D.J. Hunter, S. Lindström, and F. Canzian. 2011. Interactions between genetic variants and breast cancer risk factors in the breast and prostate cancer cohort consortium. J. Natl. Cancer Inst. 103(16):1252-1263.

Campo, E., S.H. Swerdlow, N.L. Harris, S. Pileri, H. Stein and E.S. Jaffe. 2011. The 2008 WHO classification of lymphoid neoplasms and beyond: Evolving concepts and practical applications. Blood 117(19):5019-5032.

Cardarelli, R., K.M. Cardarelli, K.G. Fulda, A. Espinoza, C. Cage, J. Vishwanatha, R. Young, D.N. Steele, and J. Carroll. 2010. Self-reported racial discrimination, response to unfair treatment, and coronary calcification in asymptomatic adults: The North Texas Healthy Heart study. BMC Public Health 10:285.

Caspi, A., A.R. Hariri, A. Holmes, R. Uher, and T.E. Moffitt. 2010. Genetic sensitivity to the environment: The case of the serotonin transporter gene and its implications for studying complex diseases and traits. Am. J. Psychiatry 167(5):509-527.

CDC (Centers for Disease Control and Prevention). 2010. Exposome and Exposomics. Centers for Disease Control and Prevention [online]. Available: http://www.cdc.gov/niosh/topics/exposome/ [accessed July 29, 2011].

CDC (Centers for Disease Control and Prevention). 2011. Social Determinants of Health. Centers for Disease Control and Prevention [online]. Available: http://www.cdc.gov/socialdeterminants/ [accessed July 29, 2011].

Chen, E., G.E. Miller, H.A. Walker, J.M. Arevalo, C.Y. Sung, and S.W. Cole. 2009. Genome-wide transcriptional profiling linked to social class in asthma. Thorax 64(1):38-43.

Cheong, H.S., S.M. Park, M.O. Kim, J.S. Park, J.Y. Lee, J.Y. Byun, B.L. Park, H.D. Shin, and C.S. Park. 2011. Genome-wide methylation profile of nasal polyps: Relation to aspirin hypersensitivity in asthmatics. Allergy 66(5):637-644.

Chute, C.G. 2011. ICD-11 and Next Generation of Clinical Classification. Presentation at NAS Framework for Developing a New Taxonomy of Disease, March 1, 2011, Washington, DC.

Cole, S.W., L.C. Hawkley, J.M. Arevalo, C.Y. Sung, R.M. Rose, and J.T. Cacioppo. 2007. Social regulation of gene expression in human leukocytes. Genome Biol. 8(9):R189.

Collins, F.S. 2004. The case for a U.S. prospective cohort study of genes and environment. Nature 429(6990):475-477.

Cornelis, M.C., A. Agrawal, J.W. Cole, N.N. Hansel, K.C. Barnes, T.H. Beaty, S.N. Bennett, L.J. Bierut, E. Boerwinkle, K.F. Doheny, B. Feenstra, E. Feingold, M. Fornage, C.A. Haiman, E.L. Harris, M.G. Hayes, J.A. Heit, F.B. Hu, J.H. Kang, C.C. Laurie, H. Ling, T.A. Manolio, M.L. Marazita, R.A. Mathias, D.B. Mirel, J. Paschall, L.R. Pasquale, E.W. Pugh, J.P. Rice, J. Udren, R.M. van Dam, X. Wang, J.L. Wiggs, K. Williams, and K. Yu; GENEVA Consortium. 2010. The Gene, Environment Association studies consortium (GENEVA): Maximizing the knowledge obtained from GWAS by collaboration across studies of multiple conditions. Genet. Epidemiol. 34(4):364-372.

Cutts, D.B., A.F. Meyers, M.M. Black, P.H. Casey, M. Chilton, J.T. Cook, J. Geppert, S. Ettinger de Cuba, T. Heeren, S. Coleman, R. Rose-Jacobs, and D.A. Frank. 2011. U.S. housing insecurity and the health of very young children. Am. J. Public Health 101(8):1508-1514.

D'Acremont, V., C. Lengeler, H. Mshinda, D. Mtasiwa, M. Tanner, and B. Genton. 2009. Time to move from presumptive malaria treatment to laboratory-confirmed diagnosis and treatment in African children with fever. PLoS Med. 6(1):e252.

Damschroder, L.J., J.L. Pritts, M.A. Neblo, R.J. Kalarickal, J.W. Creswell, and R.A. Hayward. 2007. Patients, privacy and trust: Patients' willingness to allow researchers to access their medical records. Soc. Sci. Med. 64(1):223-235.

Denny, J.C., M.D. Ritchie, M.A. Basford, J.M. Pulley, L. Bastarache, K. Brown-Gentry, D. Wang, D.R. Masys, D.M. Roden, and D.C. Crawford. 2010. PheWAS: Demonstrating the feasibility of a phenome-wide scan to discover gene-disease associations. Bioinformatics 26(9):1205-1210.

DHHS (U.S. Department of Health and Human Services). 2010. Tobacco Smoke Causes Disease: The Biology and Behavioral Basis for Smoking-Attributable Disease. A Report of the Surgeon General, U.S. Department of Health and Human Services, Public Health Service, Rockville, MD [online]. Available: http://www.surgeongeneral.gov/library/tobaccosmoke/report/index.html [accessed July 29, 2011].

Epel, E.S., E.H. Blackburn, J. Lin, F.S. Dhabhar, N.E. Adler, J.D. Morrow, and R.M. Cawthon. 2004. Accelerated telomere shortening in response to life stress. Proc. Natl. Acad. Sci. USA 101(49):17312-17315.

ESRI (Environmental Systems Research Institute, Inc.). 1990. Pp. 1-2 in Understanding GIS: The ARC/INFO Method. Redlands, CA: ESRI.

Fackenthal, J.D., and O.I. Olopade. 2007. Breast cancer risk associated with BRCA1 and BRCA2 in diverse populations. Nat. Rev. Cancer 7(12):937-948.

Fajans, S.S., G.I. Bell, and K.S. Polonsky. 2001. Molecular mechanisms and clinical pathophysiology of maturity-onset diabetes of the young. N. Engl. J. Med. 345(13):971-980.

Favello, A., L. Hillier, and R.K. Wilson. 1995. Genomic DNA sequencing methods. Methods Cell Biol. 48:551-569.

Flexner, A. 1910. Medical Education in the United States and Canada. New York: The Carnegie Foundation.

FPA (Fire Program Analysis). 2011. GIS Overview. FPA Project, Idaho State Office, BLM, Boise, ID [online]. Available: http://www.fpa.nifc.gov/Library/Documentation/FPA_PM_ Reference_Information/Output/GIS_overview.html {accessed August 19, 2011].

Franks, P.W., S. Bhattacharyya, J. Luan, C. Montague, J. Brennand, B. Challis, S. Brage, U. Ekelund, R.P. Middelberg, S. O'Rahilly, and N.J. Wareham. 2004. Association between physical activity and blood pressure is modified by variants in the G-protein coupled receptor 10. Hypertension 43(2):224-228.

Gayther, S.A., W. Warren, S. Mazoyer, P.A. Russell, P.A. Harrington, M. Chiano, S. Seal, R. Hamoudi, E.J. van Rensburg, A.M. Dunning, R. Love, G. Evans, D. Easton, D. Clayton, M.R. Stratton, and B.A. Ponder. 1995. Germline mutations of the BRCA1 gene in breast and ovarian cancer families provide evidence for a genotype-phenotype correlation. Nat. Genet. 11(4):428-433.

Ge, D., J. Fellay, A.J. Thompson, J.S. Simon, K.V. Shianna, T.J. Urban, E.L. Heinzen, P. Qiu, A.H. Bertelsen, A.J. Muir, M. Sulkowski, J.G. McHutchison, and D.B. Goldstein. 2009. Genetic variation in IL28B predicts hepatitis C treatment-induced viral clearance. Nature 461(7262):399-401.

Goh, K.I., M.E. Cusick, D. Valle, B. Childs, M. Vidal, and A.L. Barabási. 2007. The human disease network. Proc. Natl. Acad. Sci. USA 104(21):8685-8690.

Gordon, S. 2011. Metformin still best first-line type 2 diabetes drug. U.S. News Health, March 14, 2011 [online]. Available: ttp://health.usnews.com/health-news/diet-fitness/diabetes/ articles/2011/03/14/metformin-still-best-first-line-type-2-diabetes-drug [accessed October 4, 2011].

Gravlee, C.C. 2009. How race becomes biology: Embodiment of social inequality. Am. J. Phys. Anthropol. 139(1):47-57.

Greely, H.T. 2007. The uneasy ethical and legal underpinnings of large-scale genomic biobanks. Annu. Rev. Genomics Hum. Genet. 8:343-364.

Guisti, K. 2011. Presentation at NAS Framework for Developing a New Taxonomy of Disease, March 1, 2011, Washington, DC.

Haga, S.B, and J. O'Daniel. 2011. Public perspectives regarding data-sharing practices in genomics research. Public Health Genomics 14(6):319-324.

Hall, M.A., N.M. King, L.H. Perdue, J.E. Hilner, B. Akolkar, C.J. Greenbaum, and C. McKeon. 2010. Biobanking, consent, and commercialization in international genetics research: The Type 1 Diabetes Genetics Consortium. Clin. Trials 7(suppl. 1):S33-S45.

HealthyPeople.gov. 2011. Healthy People 2020 [online]. Available: http://www.healthypeople. gov/2020/about/DOHAbout.aspx [accessed July 28, 2011].

Hill, T.D., L.M. Graham, and V. Divgi. 2011. Racial disparities in pediatric asthma: A review of the literature. Curr. Allergy Asthma Rep. 11(1):85-90.

Hu, F.B., and V.S. Malik. 2010. Sugar-sweetened beverages and risk of obesity and type 2 diabetes: Epidemiologic evidence. Physiol. Behav. 100(1):47-54.

Hudson, K.L., M.K. Holohan, and F.S. Collins. 2008. Keeping pace with the times—the Genetic Information Nondiscrimination Act of 2008. N. Engl. J. Med. 358(25):2661-2663.

Huijgen, R., M.N. Vissers, J.C. Defesche, P.J. Lansberg, J.J. Kastelein, and B.A. Hutten. 2008. Familial hypercholesterolemia: Current treatment and advances in management. Expert Rev. Cardiovasc. Ther. 6(4):567-581.

IOM (Institute of Medicine). 2006. Genes, Behavior, and the Social Environment: Moving Beyond the Nature/Nurture Debate. Washington, DC: National Academies Press.

IOM (Institute of Medicine). 2009. Beyond the HIPAA Privacy Rule: Enhancing Privacy, Improving Health through Research, S. Nass, L. Leavitt, and L. Gostin, eds. Washington, DC: National Academies Press.

IOM (Institute of Medicine). 2010a. Challenges and Opportunities in Using Residual Newborn Screening Samples for Translational Research. Washington, DC: National Academies Press.

IOM (Institute of Medicine). 2010b. Extending the Spectrum of Precompetitive Collaboration in Oncology Research: Workshop Summary, M. Patlack, S. Nass, E. Balogh, eds. Washington, DC: National Academies Press.

IOM (Institute of Medicine). 2011. Establishing Precompetitive Collaborations to Simulate Genomics-Driven Drug Development: Workshop Summary. Washington, DC: National Academies Press.

Jones, R., M. Pembrey, J. Golding, and D. Herrick. 2005. The search for genenotype/phenotype associations and the phenome scan. Paediatr. Perinat. Epidemiol. 19(4):264-265.

Kaaks, R., S. Rinaldi, T.J. Key, F. Berrino, P.H. Peeters, C. Biessy, L. Dossus, A. Lukanova, S. Bingham, K.T. Khaw, N.E. Allen, H.B. Bueno-de-Mesquita, C.H. van Gils, D. Grobbee, H. Boeing, P.H. Lahmann, G. Nagel, J. Chang-Claude, F. Clavel-Chapelon, A. Fournier, A. Thiébaut, C.A. González, J.R. Quirós, M.J. Tormo, E. Ardanaz, P. Amiano, V. Krogh, D. Palli, S. Panico, R. Tumino, P. Vineis, A. Trichopoulou, V. Kalapothaki, D. Trichopoulos, P. Ferrari, T. Norat, R. Saracci, and E. Riboli. 2005. Postmenopausal serum androgens, oestrogens and breast cancer risk: The European prospective investigation into cancer and nutrition. Endocr. Relat. Cancer 12(4):1071-1082.

Karelina, K., and A.C. DeVries. 2011. Modeling social influences on human health. Psychosom. Med. 73(1):67-74.

Kellett, A. 2011. Diabetes Mellitus Type 2. Virtual Care Health Team, School of Health Professions at the University of Missouri-Columbia [online]. Available: http://www.vhct.org/case2600/index.htm [accessed October 4, 2011].

Kho, A.N., J.A. Pacheco, P.L. Peissig, L. Rasmussen, K.M. Newton, N. Weston, P.K. Crane, J. Pathak, C.G. Chute, S.J. Bielinski, I.J. Kullo, R. Li, T.A. Manolio, R.L. Chisholm, and J.C. Denny. 2011. Electronic medical records for genetic research: Results of the eMERGE consortium. Sci. Transl. Med. 3(79):79re1.

Khoury, M., and S. Wacholder. 2009. Invited commentary: From genome-wide association studies to gene-environment-wide interaction studies--Challenges and opportunities. Am. J. Epidemiol.169(2):227-230.

Kim, D., K.E. Masyn, I. Kawachi, F. Laden, and G.A. Colditz. 2010. Neighborhood socioeconomic status and behavioral pathways to risks of colon and rectal cancer in women. Cancer 116(17):4187-4196.

King, M.C., J.H. Marks, J.B. Mandell, and the New York Breast Cancer Study Group. 2003. Breast and ovarian cancer risks due to inherited mutations in BRCA1 and BRCA2. Science 302(5645):643-646.

Kiyoi, H., T. Naoe, Y. Nakano, S. Yokota, S. Minami, S. Miyawaki, N. Asou, K. Kuriyama, I. Jinnai, C. Shimazaki, H. Akiyama, K. Saito, H. Oh, T. Motoji, E. Omoto, H. Saito, R. Ohno, and R. Ueda. 1999. Prognostic implication of FLT3 and N-RAS gene mutations in acute myeloid leukemia. Blood 93(9):3074-3080.

Klecka, G., C. Persoon, and R. Currie. 2010. Chemicals of emerging concern in the Great Lakes Basin: An analysis of environmental exposures. Rev. Environ. Contam. Toxicol. 207:1-93.

Kolata, G. 2011. How Bright Promise in Cancer Testing Fell Apart. New York Times, July 8, 2011[online]. Available: http://www.nytimes.com/2011/07/08/health/research/08genes.html [accessed August 4, 2011].

Kottaridis, P.D., R.E. Gale, M.E. Frew, G. Harrison, S.E. Langabeer, A.A. Belton, H. Walker, K. Wheatley, D.T. Bowen, A.K. Burnett, A.H. Goldstone, and D.C. Linch. 2001. The presence of a FLT3 internal tandem duplication in patients with acute myeloid leukemia (AML) adds important prognostic information to cytogenetic risk group and response to the first cycle of chemotherapy: Analysis of 854 patients from the United Kingdom Medical Research Council AML 10 and 12 trials. Blood 98(6):1752-1759.

Krieger, N., J.T. Chen, B.A. Coull, and J.V. Selby. 2005. Lifetime socioeconomic position and twins' health: An analysis of 308 pairs of United States women twins. PLoS Med. 2(7):e162.

Kris, M.G., R.B. Natale, R.S. Herbst, T.J. Lynch, Jr., D. Prager, C.P. Belani, J.H. Schiller, K. Kelly, H. Spiridonidis, A. Sandler, K.S. Albain, D. Cella, M.K. Wolf, S.D. Averbuch, J.J. Ochs, and A.C. Kay. 2003. Efficacy of gefitinib, an inhibitor of the epidermal growth factor receptor tyrosine kinase, in symptomatic patients with non-small cell lung cancer: A randomized trial. JAMA 290(16):2149-2158.

Kwak, E.L., Y.J. Bang, D.R. Camidge, A.T. Shaw, B. Solomon, R.G. Maki, S.H. Ou, B.J. Dezube, P.A. Jänne, D.B. Costa, M. Varella-Garcia, W.H. Kim, T.J. Lynch, P. Fidias, H. Stubbs, J.A. Engelman, L.V. Sequist, W. Tan, L. Gandhi, M. Mino-Kenudson, G.C. Wei, S.M. Shreeve, M.J. Ratain, J. Settleman, J.G. Christensen, D.A. Haber, K. Wilner, R. Salgia, G.I. Shapiro, J.W. Clark, and A.J. Iafrate. 2010. Anaplastic lymphoma kinase inhibition in non-small-cell lung cancer. N. Engl. J. Med. 363(18):1693-1703.

Lee, S.H., J.S. Park, and C.S. Park. 2011. The search for genetic variants and epigenetics related to asthma. Allergy Asthma Immunol. Res. 3(4):236-244.

Levy, D., G.L. Splansky, N.K. Strand, L.D. Atwood, E.J. Benjamin, S. Blease, L.A. Cupples, R.B. D'Agostino, Sr., C.S. Fox, M. Kelly-Hayes, G. Koski, M.G. Larson, K.M. Mutalik, E. Oberacker, C.J. O'Donnell, P. Sutherland, M. Valentino, R.S. Vasan, P.A. Wolf, and J.M. Murabito. 2010. Consent for genetic research in the Framingham Heart Study. Am. J. Med. Genet. A. 152A(5):1250-1256.

Li, X., T.D. Howard, S.L. Zheng, T. Haselkorn, S.P. Peters, D.A. Meyers, and E.R. Bleecker. 2010. Genome-wide association study of asthma identifies RAD50-IL13 and HLA-DR/DQ regions. J. Allergy Clin. Immunol. 125(2):328-35.e11.

Linné, C.V. 1763. *Genera morborum*. Uppsala: Steinert [online]. Available: http://gallica.bnf.fr/ [accessed August 3, 2011].

Lorsch, J.R. 2011. Potential Impact of a New Taxonomy of Disease on Medical and Graduate Biomedical Education.

Lorsch, J.R., and D.G. Nichols. 2011. Organizing graduate life sciences education around nodes and connections. Cell 146(4):506-509.

Loscalzo, J., I. Kohane, and A.L. Barabasi. 2007. Human disease classification in the postgenomic era: A complex systems approach to human pathobiology. Mol. Syst. Biol. 3:124.

Lynch, T.J., D.W. Bell, R. Sordella, S. Gurubhagavatula, R.A. Okimoto, B.W. Brannigan, P.L. Harris, S.M. Haserlat, J.G. Supko, F.G. Haluska, D.N. Louis, D.C. Christiani, J. Settleman, and D.A. Haber. 2004. Activating mutations in the epidermal growth factor receptor underlying responsiveness of non-small-cell lung cancer to gefitinib. N. Engl. J. Med. 350(21):2129-2139.

malERA Consultative Group on Diagnoses and Diagnostics. 2011. A research agenda for malaria eradication: Diagnoses and diagnostics. PLoS Med. 8(1):e1000396.

Malone, K.E., J.R. Daling, D.R. Doody, L. Hsu, L. Bernstein, R.J. Coates, P.A. Marchbanks, M.S. Simon, J.A. McDonald, S.A. Norman, B.L. Strom, R.T. Burkman, G. Ursin, D. Deapen, L.K. Weiss, S. Folger, J.J. Madeoy, D.M. Friedrichsen, N.M. Suter, M.C. Humphrey, R. Spirtas, and E.A. Ostrander. 2006. Prevalence and predictors of BRCA1 and BRCA2 mutations in a population-based study of breast cancer in white and black American women ages 35 to 64 years. Cancer Res. 66(16):8297-8308.

Mardis, E.R. 2011. A decade's perspective on DNA sequencing technology. Nature 470(7333): 198-203.

Masys, D. 2011. Extracting Phenotypes from EMRs for Genetic Association Studies: The eMERGE Consortium Experience and Implications for New Taxonomies. Presentation at NAS Framework for Developing a New Taxonomy of Disease, March 2, 2011, Washington, DC.

Maxam, A.M., and W. Gilbert. 1977. A new method for sequencing DNA. Proc. Natl. Acad. Sci. USA. 74(2):560-564.

McCarthy, M.I., G.R. Abecasis, L.R. Cardon, D.B. Goldstein, J. Little, J.P. Ioannidis, and J.N. Hirschhorn. 2008. Genome-wide association studies for complex traits: Consensus, uncertainty and challenges. Nat. Rev. Genet. 9(5):356-369.

McCarty, C.A., R.L. Chisholm, C.G. Chute, I. Kullo, G. Jarvik, E.B. Larson, R. Li, D.R. Masys, M.D. Ritchie, D.M. Roden, J. Struewing, and W.A.Wolf. 2011. The eMERGE Network: A consortium of biorepositories linked to electronic medical records data for conducting genomic studies. BMC Med. Genomics 4:13.

McGuire, A.L., M. Basford, L.G. Dressler, S.M. Fullerton, B.A. Koenig, R. Li, C.A. McCarty, E. Ramos, M.E. Smith, C.P. Somkin, C. Waudby, W.A. Wolf, and E.W. Clayton. 2011. Ethical and practical challenges of sharing data from genome-wide association studies: The eMERGE Consortium experience. Genome Res. 21(7):1001-1007.

McMichael, A.J., and E. Lindgren. 2011. Climate change: Present and future risks to health, and necessary responses. J. Intern. Med. 270(5)"401-413.

Missmer, S.A., A.H. Eliassen, R.L. Barbieri, and S.E. Hankinson. 2004. Endogenous estrogen, androgen, and progesterone concentrations and breast cancer risk among postmenopausal women. J. Natl. Cancer Inst. 96(24):1856-1865.

MIT (Massachusetts Institute of Technology). 2011. The Third Revolution: The Convergence of the Life Sciences, Physical Sciences, and Engineering. Massachusetts Institute of Technology [online]. Available: http://web.mit.edu/dc/policy/MIT%20White%20Paper%20on%20 Convergence.pdf [accessed August 5, 2011].

MITRE Corporation. 2010. The $100 Genome: Implications for the DoD. JSR-10-100. JASON Program Office, MITRE Corporation, McLean, VA. December 2010 [online]. Available: http://www.fas.org/irp/agency/dod/jason/hundred.pdf [accessed August 3, 2011].

Moffatt, M.F., I.G. Gut, F. Demenais, D.P. Strachan, E. Bouzigon, S. Heath, E. von Mutius, M. Farrall, M. Lathrop, and W.O. Cookson. 2010. A large-scale, consortium-based genomewide association study of asthma. N. Engl. J. Med. 363(13):1211-1221.

MSKCC (Memorial Sloan-Kettering Cancer Center). 2005. Why Some Lung Cancers Stop Responding to Tarceva and Iressa. EurekAlert. Org., February 21, 2005 [online]. Available: http://www.eurekalert.org/pub_releases/2005-02/mscc-wsl021605.php [accessed August 19, 2011].

Munos, B. 2009. Lessons from 60 years of pharmaceutical innovation. Nat. Rev. Drug Discov. 8(12):959-968.

Murcray, C.E., J.P. Lewinger, and W.J. Gauderman. 2009. Gene-environment interaction in genome-wide association studies. Am. J. Epidemiol. 169(2):219-226.

NAS (The National Academies). 2010. The Exposome: A Powerful Approach for Evaluating Environmental Exposures and Their Influences on Human Disease. The Newsletter of the Standing Committee on Use of Emerging Science for Environmental Health Decisions. June 2010 [online]. Available: http://dels-old.nas.edu/envirohealth/newsletters/newsletter3_exposomes.pdf [accessed July 29, 2011].

NCBI (National Center for Biotechnology Information). 2011a. Growth of GenBank. GenBank Statistics, National Center for Biotechnology Information [online]. Available: http://www.ncbi.nlm.nih.gov/genbank/genbankstats.html [accessed April 29, 2011].

NCBI (National Center for Biotechnology Information). 2011b. dbGap: Database of Genotypes and Phenotypes. National Center for Biotechnology Information [online]. Available: http://www.ncbi.nlm.nih.gov/gap [accessed August 5, 2011].

Need, A.C., and D.B. Goldstein. 2009. Next generation disparities in human genomics: Concerns and remedies. Trends Genet. 25(11):489-494.

Ng, S.B., E.H. Turner, P.D. Robertson, S.D. Flygare, A.W. Bigham, C. Lee, T. Shaffer, M. Wong, A. Bhattacharjee, E.E. Eichler, M. Bamshad, D.A. Nickerson, and J. Shendure. 2009. Targeted capture and massively parallel sequencing of 12 human exomes. Nature 461(7261):272-276.

NHGRI (National Human Genome Research Institute). 2011. BIC Database of BRCA1 Mutations. National Human Genome Research Institute [online]. Available: http://www.research.nhgri.nih.gov/projects/bic/Member/brca1_mutation_database.shtml [accessed April 30, 2011].

NRC (National Research Council). 2009. A New Biology for the 21st Century. Washington, DC: National Academies Press.

Nunez, M., A.M. Saran, and B.I. Freedman. 2010. Gene-gene and gene-environment interactions in HIV-associated nephropathy: A focus on the MYH9 nephropathy susceptibility gene. Adv. Chronic Kidney Dis. 17(1):44-51.

OECD (Organization for Economic Co-operation and Development). 2011. OECD Health Data. Organization for Economic Co-operation and Development [online]. Available: http://www.oecd.org/document/30/0,3746,en_2649_37407_12968734_1_1_1_37407,00.html [accessed August 3, 2011].

Paez, J.G., P.A. Jänne, J.C. Lee, S. Tracy, H. Greulich, S. Gabriel, P. Herman, F.J. Kaye, N. Lindeman, T.J. Boggon, K. Naoki, H. Sasaki, Y. Fujii, M.J. Eck, W.R. Sellers, B.E. Johnson, and M. Meyerson. 2004. EGFR mutations in lung cancer: Correlation with clinical response to gefitinib therapy. Science 304(5676):1497-1500.

Palmer, L.J. 2007. UK biobank: Bank on it. Lancet 369(9578):1980-1982.

Pao, W., and N. Girard. 2011. New driver mutations in non-small-cell lung cancer. Lancet Oncol. 12(2):175-180.

Pao, W., and V.A. Miller. 2005. Epidermal growth factor receptor mutations, small-molecule kinase inhibitors, and non-small-cell lung cancer: Current knowledge and future directions. J. Clin. Oncol. 23(11):2556-2568.

Pao, W., V. Miller, M. Zakowski, J. Doherty, K. Politi, I. Sarkaria, B. Singh, R. Heelan, V. Rusch, L. Fulton, E. Mardis, D. Kupfer, R. Wilson, M. Kris, and H. Varmus. 2004. EGF receptor gene mutations are common in lung cancers from "never smokers" and are associated with sensitivity of tumors to gefitinib and erlotinib. Proc. Natl. Acad. Sci. USA 101(36):13306-13311.

PatientsLikeMe.com. 2011. Treatment and Side Effect from Patient Like You [online]. Available: http://www.patientslikeme.com/ [accessed October 8, 2011].

PCAST (President's Council of Advisors on Science and Technology). 2008. Priorities for Personalized Medicine. President's Council of Advisors on Science and Technology, September 2008 [online]. Available: http://www.whitehouse.gov/files/documents/ostp/PCAST/pcast_report_v2.pdf [accessed August 3, 2011].

PCAST (President's Council of Advisors on Science and Technology). 2010. Report to the President. Realizing the Full Potential of Health Information Technology to Improve Health Care for Americans: The Path Forward. Executive Office of the President, President's Council of Advisors on Science and Technology [online]. Available: http://www.whitehouse.gov/sites/default/files/microsites/ostp/pcast-health-it-report.pdf [accessed September 22, 2011]

Pelak, K., K.V. Shianna, D. Ge, J.M. Maia, M. Zhu, J.P. Smith, E.T. Cirulli, J. Fellay, S.P. Dickson, C.E. Gumbs, E.L. Heinzen, A.C. Need, E.K. Ruzzo, A. Singh, C.R. Campbell, L.K. Hong, K.A. Lornsen, A.M. McKenzie, N.L. Sobreira, J.E. Hoover-Fong, J.D. Milner, R. Ottman, B.F. Haynes, J.J. Goedert, and D.B. Goldstein. 2010. The characterization of twenty sequenced human genomes. PLoS Genet. 6(9):e1001111.

Pollack, C.E., B.A. Griffin, and J. Lynch. 2010. Housing affordability and health among homeowners and renters. Am. J. Prev. Med. 39(6):515-521.

PRNewswire. 2011. Quest Diagnostics Launches Hepatitis C Virus Therapy Test Based on IL28B Gene Variants: AccuType® IL28B Test Now Available to Physicians and for Clinical Trials Research. PRNewswire, April 18, 2011 [online]. Available: http://www.prnewswire.com/news-releases/quest-diagnostics-launches-hepatitis-c-virus-therapy-test-based-on-il28b-gene-variants-120056609.html [accessed August 2, 2011].

Pulley, J., E. Clayton, G.R. Bernard, D.M. Roden, and D.R. Masys. 2010. Principles of human subjects protections applied in an opt-out, de-identified biobank. Clin. Transl. Sci. 3(1):42-48.

Quinn, K., J.S. Kaufman, A. Siddiqi, and K. Yeatts. 2010. Stress and the city: Housing stressors are associated with respiratory health among low socioeconomic status Chicago children. J. Urban Health 87(4):688-702.

Rappaport, S.M. 2011. Implications of the exposome for exposure science. J. Expo. Sci. Environ. Epidemiol. 21(1):5-9.

Roden, D.M., J.M. Pulley, M.A. Basford, G.R. Bernard, E.W. Clayton, J.R. Balser, and D.R. Masys. 2008. Development of a large-scale de-identified DNA biobank to enable personalized medicine. Clin. Pharmacol. Ther. 84(3):362-369.

Roukos, D.H., and E. Briasoulis. 2007. Individualized preventive and therapeutic management of hereditary breast ovarian cancer syndrome. Nat. Clin. Pract. Oncol. 4(10):578-590.

Ryu, E., B.L. Fridley, N. Tosakulwong, K.R. Bailey, and A.O. Edwards. 2010. Genome-wide association analyses of genetic, phenotypic, and environmental risks in the age-related eye disease study. Mol Vis. 16:2811-2821.

Sanger, F., S. Nicklen, and A.R. Coulson. 1977. DNA sequencing with chain-terminating inhibitors. Proc. Natl. Acad. Sci. USA 74(12):5463-5467.

Sankaran, V.G., T.F. Menne, J. Xu, T.E. Akie, G. Lettre, B. Van Handel, H.K. Mikkola, J.N. Hirschhorn, A.B. Cantor, and S.H. Orkin. 2008. Human fetal hemoglobin expression is regulated by the developmental stage-specific repressor BCL11A. Science 322(5909):1839-1842.

Scripps Health. 2011. IL28B Genetic Testing to Hepatitis C Patients Now Available. New HCV Drug, February 25, 2011 [online]. Available: http://hepatitiscnewdrugs.blogspot.com/2011/02/scripps-health-il28b-genetic-testing-to.html[accessed August 1, 2011].

Searing, D.A., Y. Zhang, J.R. Murphy, P.J. Hauk, E. Goleva, and D.Y. Leung. 2010. Decreased serum vitamin D levels in children with asthma are associated with increased corticosteroid use. J. Allergy Clin. Immunol. 125(5):995-1000.

Siemens Healthcare Diagnostics Inc. 2008. Breast Cancer Case Study. Siemens Healthcare Diagnostics Inc., Deerfield, IL [online]. Available: http://www.medical.siemens.com/siemens/en_GLOBAL/gg_diag_FBAs/files/Assays/HER2_neu/0701095_BreastCancerCaseStudy.pdf [accessed October 4, 2011].

Small, P.M., and M. Pai. 2010. Tuberculosis diagnosis—time for a game change. N. Engl. J. Med. 363(11):1070-1071.

Smith, A.M., D.I. Bernstein, G.K. LeMasters, N.L. Huey, M. Ericksen, M. Villareal, J. Lockey, and G.K. Khurana Hershey. 2008. Environmental tobacco smoke and interleukin 4 polymorphism (C-589T) gene: Environment interaction increases risk of wheezing in African-American infants. J. Pediatr. 152(5):709-715.

Snieder, H., G.A. Harshfield, P. Barbeau, D.M. Pollock, J.S. Pollock, and F.A. Treiber. 2002. Dissecting the genetic architecture of the cardiovascular and renal stress response. Biol. Psychol. 61(1-2):73-95.

Soda, M., Y.L. Choi, M. Enomoto, S. Takada, Y. Yamashita, S. Ishikawa, S. Fujiwara, H. Watanabe, K. Kurashina, H. Hatanaka, M. Bando, S. Ohno, Y. Ishikawa, H. Aburatani, T. Niki, Y. Sohara, Y. Sugiyama, and H. Mano. 2007. Identification of the transforming EML4-ALK fusion gene in non-small-cell lung cancer. Nature 448(7153):561-566.

Sternthal, M.J., B.A. Coull, Y.H. Mathilda Chiu, S. Cohen, and R.J. Wright. 2011. Associations among maternal childhood socioeconomic status, cord blood IgE levels, and repeated wheeze in urban children. J. Allergy Clin. Immunol. 128(2):337-345.e1.

Sweetenham, J.W. 2011. Molecular signatures in the diagnosis and management of diffuse large B-cell lymphoma. Curr. Opin. Hematol. 18(4):288-292.

Travis, W.D., E. Brambilla, M. Noguchi, A.G. Nicholson, K.R. Geisinger, Y. Yatabe, D.G. Beer, C.A. Powell, G.J. Riely, P.E. Van Schil, K. Garg, J.H. Austin, H. Asamura, V.W. Rusch, F.R. Hirsch, G. Scagliotti, T. Mitsudomi, R.M. Huber, Y. Ishikawa, J. Jett, M. Sanchez-Cespedes, J.P. Sculier, T. Takahashi, M. Tsuboi, J. Vansteenkiste, I. Wistuba, P.C. Yang, D. Aberle, C. Brambilla, D. Flieder, W. Franklin, A. Gazdar, M. Gould, P. Hasleton, D. Henderson, B. Johnson, D. Johnson, K. Kerr, K. Kuriyama, J.S. Lee, V.A. Miller, I. Petersen, V. Roggli, R. Rosell, N. Saijo, E. Thunnissen, M. Tsao, and D. Yankelewitz. 2011. International association for the study of lung cancer/American Thoracic Society/European Respiratory Society international multidisciplinary classification of lung adenocarcinoma. J. Thorac. Oncol. 6(2):244-285.

Trinidad, S.B., S.M. Fullerton, J.M. Bares, G.P. Jarvik, E.B. Larson, and W. Burke. 2010. Genomic research and wide data sharing: Views of prospective participants. Genet. Med. 12(8):486-495.

Trinidad, S.B., S.M. Fullerton, E.J. Ludman, G.P. Jarvik, E.B. Larson, and W. Burke. 2011. Research ethics. Research practice and participant preferences: The growing gulf. Science 331(6015):287-288.

Tu, S.W., O. Bodenreider, C. Çelik, C.G. Chute, S. Heard, R. Jakob, G. Jiang, S. Kim, E. Miller, M.M. Musen, J. Nakaya, J. Patrick, A. Rector, G. Reynoso, J.M. Rodrigues, H. Solbrig, K.A Spackman, T. Tudorache, S. Weber, and T.B. Üstün. 2010. A Content Model for the ICD-11 Revision. BMIR-2010-1405. Stanford Center for Biomedical Informatics Research [online]. Available: .http://bmir.stanford.edu/file_asset/index.php/1522/BMIR-2010-1405.pdf [accessed October 5, 2011].

Turnbaugh, P.J., R.E. Ley, M.Hamady, C.M. Fraser-Liggett, R. Knight, and J.I. Gordon. 2007. The human microbiome project. Nature 449(7164):804-810.

UnnaturalCauses.org. 2008. Unnatural Causes [online]. http://www.unnaturalcauses.org. [accessed August 1, 2011].

Vardiman, J.W., J. Thiele, D.A. Arber, R.D. Brunning, M.J. Borowitz, A. Porwit, N.L. Harris, M.M. Le Beau, E. Hellstrom-Lindberg, A. Tefferi, and C.D. Bloomfield. 2009. The 2008 revision of the World Health Organization (WHO) classification of myeloid neoplasms and acute leukemia: Rationale and important changes. Blood 114(5):937-951.

Vargas, G., B. Boutouyrie, S. Ostrowitzki, and L. Santarelli. 2010. Arguments against precompetitive collaboration. Clin. Pharmacol. Ther. 87(5):527-529.

Wang, T.J., M.G. Larson, R.S. Vasan, S. Cheng, E.P. Rhee, E. McCabe, G.D. Lewis, C.S. Fox, P.F. Jacques, C. Fernandez, C.J. O'Donnell, S.A. Carr, V.K. Mootha, J.C. Florez, A. Souza, O. Melander, C.B. Clish, and R.E. Gerszten. 2011. Metabolite profiles and the risk of developing diabetes. Nat. Med. 17(4):448-453.

Wetterstrand, K.A. 2011. DNA Sequencing Costs: Data from the NHGRI Large-Scale Genome Sequencing Program [online]. Available http://www.genome.gov/sequencingcosts/ [accessed June 18, 2011].

WHO (World Health Organization). 2007. International Statistical Classification of Diseases and Related Health Problems, 10th Revision. Geneva: World Health Organization [online] http://apps.who.int/classifications/apps/icd/icd10online/ [accessed August 3, 2011].

WHO (World Health Organization). 2011. Social Determinants of Health: Key Concepts World Health Organization [online]. Available: http://www.who.int/social_determinants/thecommission/finalreport/key_concepts/en/index.html [accessed August 1, 2011].

Wiener, C.M., P.A. Thomas, E. Goodspeed, D. Valle, and D.G. Nichols. 2010. "Genes to society"—the logic and process of the new curriculum for the Johns Hopkins University School of Medicine. Acad. Med. 85(3):498-506.

Wilbur, C.L. 1911. Manual of the International List of Causes of Death, 2nd Revision. Washington, DC: U.S. Government Printing Office.

Wild, C.P. 2005. Complementing the genome with an "exposome": The outstanding challenge of environmental exposure measurement in molecular epidemiology. Cancer Epidemiol. Biomarkers Prev. 14(8):1847-1850.

Willett, W.C., W.J. Blot, G.A. Colditz, A.R. Folsom, B.E. Henderson, and M.J. Stampfer. 2007. Merging and emerging cohorts: Not worth the wait. Nature 445(7125):257-258.

Williams, D.R., and S.A. Mohammed. 2009. Discrimination and racial disparities in health: Evidence and needed research. J. Behav. Med. 32(1):20-47.

Williams, D.R., M. Sternthal, and R.J. Wright. 2009. Social determinants: Taking the social context of asthma seriously. Pediatrics 123(suppl. 3):S174-S184.

Williams, J.B., D. Pang, B. Delgado M. Kocherginsky, M. Tretiakova, T. Krausz, D. Pan, J. He, M.K. McClintock, and S.D. Conzen. 2009. A model of gene-environment interaction reveals altered mammary gland gene expression and increased tumor growth following social isolation. Cancer Prev Res.2(10):850-861.

Williams, R.B., D.A. Marchuk, K.M. Gadde, J.C. Barefoot, K. Grichnik, M.J. Helms, C.M. Kuhn, J.G. Lewis, S.M. Schanberg, M. Stafford-Smith, E.C. Suarez, G.L. Clary, I.K. Svenson, and I.C. Siegler. 2001. Central nervous system serotonin function and cardiovascular responses to stress. Psychosom. Med. 63(2):300-305.

Wolinsky, H. 2007. The thousand-dollar genome. Genetic brinkmanship or personalized medicine? EMBO Rep. 8(10):900-903.

Yorifuji, T., I. Kawachi, T. Sakamoto, and H. Doi. 2011. Associations of outdoor air pollution with hemorrhagic stroke mortality. J. Occup. Environ. Med. 53(2):124-126.

Zanobetti, A., A. Baccarelli, and J. Schwartz. 2011. Gene-air pollution interaction and cardiovascular disease: A review. Prog. Cardiovasc. Dis. 53(5):344-352.

Appendix A

The Statement of Task with Additional Context

THE NATIONAL ACADEMIES

NATIONAL ACADEMY OF SCIENCES   NATIONAL ACADEMY OF ENGINEERING
INSTITUTE OF MEDICINE   NATIONAL RESEARCH COUNCIL

DIVISION ON EARTH AND LIFE STUDIES
BOARD ON LIFE SCIENCES

PROJECT DESCRIPTION

Framework for Developing a New Taxonomy of Disease

Statement of Task

At the request of the Director's Office of NIH, an ad hoc Committee of the National Research Council will explore the feasibility and need, and develop a potential framework, for creating a "New Taxonomy" of human diseases based on molecular biology. As part of its deliberations, the Committee will host a large two-day workshop that convenes diverse experts in both basic and clinical disease biology to address the feasibility, need, scope, impact, and consequences of defining this New Taxonomy. The workshop participants will also consider the essential elements of the framework by addressing topics that include, but are not limited to:

- Compiling the huge diversity of extant data from molecular studies of human disease to assess what is known, identify gaps, and recommend priorities to fill these gaps.
- Developing effective and acceptable mechanisms and policies for selection, collection, storage, and management of data, as well as means to provide access to and interpret these data.
- Defining the roles and interfaces among the stakeholder communities—public and private funders, data contributors, clinicians, patients, industry, and others.

- Considering how to address the many ethical concerns that are likely to arise in the wake of such a program.

The Committee will also consider recommending a small number of case studies that might be used as an initial test for the framework.

The ad hoc Committee will use the workshop results in its deliberations as it develops recommendations for a framework in a consensus report. The report may form a basis for government and other research funding organizations regarding molecular studies of human disease. The report will not, however, include recommendations related to funding, government organization, or policy issues.

Project Context and Issues:

The ability to sequence genomes and transcriptomes rapidly and cheaply is producing major advances in molecular genetics. These advances, in turn, provide new tools for defining diseases by their biological mechanisms. The recognition and classification of human diseases are fundamental for the practice of medicine, with accurate diagnoses essential for successful treatment. Although diagnostics have begun to embrace the identification and measurement of molecular disease mechanisms, the classification of disease is still largely based on phenotypic factors, or "signs and symptoms." Assigning a name to a disease is not necessarily accompanied by a clear understanding of its biochemical causes or of the variations in disease manifestations among patients.

Remarkable advances in molecular biology have brought biomedical research to an "inflection point," putting the life sciences at the cusp of delivering dramatic improvements in understanding disease to reap the health benefits that formed the rationale for the Human Genome Project. In 2010, we are now poised to use genomics, proteomics, metabolomics, systems analyses, and other derivatives of molecular biology to:

- understand disease based on biochemical mechanisms rather than clinical appearances or phenotypes;
- transform disease diagnosis;
- develop improved screening for, and management of, risk factors for disease;
- discover new drugs and reduce side effects by predicting individual responses based on genetic factors; and
- transform the practice of clinical medicine.

For these benefits to be realized, however, much work remains to be done. Some in the life sciences community are calling for the launch of a wide-ranging new program to use molecular and systems approaches to build a new "taxonomy" of human diseases. The feasibility of such a program, including the readiness of the technology, willingness of the scientific community to pursue it, and compelling nature of the gaps it would fill, remains to be explored. Embarking on such a program would require that existing data linking molecular, environmental, and experiential factors to disease states be surveyed and compiled, and that gaps in these data be identified and priorities set and acted upon to fill these gaps. In addition, effective and acceptable mechanisms and policies for selection, collection, storage, and management of data, as well as perception, construction, and manipulation network relationships within the data, are clearly needed. Criteria must also be established for providing or denying access to and interpretation of data. Roles of and interfaces among the involved communities (public and private funders, data contributors, clinicians, patients, industry, and others) would need to be explored and defined. And the many ethical considerations surrounding such a program would need to be addressed.

Each of these areas is technically complex. Some are also vast, e.g., the compilation of current knowledge and the scientific research efforts needed to fill gaps. Undertaking such a program would clearly require the participation and collaboration of many government and private entities over a considerable period of time. To ensure that progress is being made, goals and milestones against which program success can be measured would need to be developed. The NIH seeks the advice of an expert NRC Committee charged with exploring the feasibility and need, and developing a framework, for a potential "New Taxonomy of Disease" effort. The Committee would leverage the expertise of additional scientists, clinicians, and others by holding a large (approximately 100 participants) workshop to obtain ideas from the broader scientific and medical communities. Following the workshop, the Committee will use the workshop results to distill its findings and recommendations for the structure and components of a framework into a consensus report to NIH. The Committee will also consider recommending a small number of case studies that might be used as an initial test for the framework.

Appendix B

Committee Biographies

COMMITTEE MEMBERS

Susan Desmond-Hellmann, M.D., M.P.H., is Chancellor of the University of California, San Francisco. She assumed the post August 3, 2009.

UCSF is a leading university dedicated to promoting health worldwide through advanced biomedical research, graduate-level education in the life sciences and health professions, and excellence in patient care. UCSF is the only campus in the 10-campus UC system devoted exclusively to the health sciences.

Dr. Desmond-Hellmann previously served as president of product development at Genentech, a position she held from March 2004 through April 30, 2009. In this role, she was responsible for Genentech's preclinical and clinical development, process research and development, business development and product portfolio management. She also served as a member of Genentech's executive Committee, beginning in 1996. She joined Genentech in 1995 as a clinical scientist, and she was named chief medical officer in 1996. In 1999, she was named executive vice president of development and product operations. During her time at Genentech, several of the company's patient therapeutics (Lucentis, Avastin, Herceptin, Tarceva, Rituxan and Xolair) were approved by the U.S. Food and Drug Administration, and the company became the nation's No. 1 producer of anti-cancer drug treatments.

She completed her clinical training at UCSF and is board-certified in internal medicine and medical oncology. She holds a bachelor of science degree in pre-medicine and a medical degree from the University of Nevada, Reno, and a master's degree in public health from the University of California, Berkeley.

Prior to joining Genentech, Dr. Desmond-Hellmann was associate director of clinical cancer research at Bristol-Myers Squibb Pharmaceutical Research

Institute. While at Bristol-Myers Squibb, she was the project team leader for the cancer-fighting drug Taxol.

Dr. Desmond-Hellmann also has served as associate adjunct professor of epidemiology and biostatistics at UCSF. During her tenure at UCSF, she spent two years as visiting faculty at the Uganda Cancer Institute, studying HIV/AIDS and cancer. She also spent two years in private practice as a medical oncologist before returning to clinical research.

In January 2009, Desmond-Hellmann joined the Federal Reserve Bank of San Francisco's Economic Advisory Council for a three-year term. In July 2008, she was appointed to the California Academy of Sciences board of trustees. Dr. Desmond-Hellmann was named to the Biotech Hall of Fame in 2007 and as the Healthcare Businesswomen's Association Woman of the Year for 2006. She was listed among *Fortune* magazine's "top 50 most powerful women in business" in 2001 and from 2003 to 2008. In 2005 and 2006, the *Wall Street Journal* listed dr. Desmond-Hellmann as one of its "women to watch." From 2005 to 2008, Dr. Desmond-Hellmann served a three-year term as a member of the American Association for Cancer Research board of directors, and from 2001 to 2009, she served on the executive committee of the board of directors of the Biotechnology Industry Organization. She served on the corporate board of Affymetrix from 2004–2009.

Charles L. Sawyers, M.D., is an Investigator of the Howard Hughes Medical Institute and the inaugural Director of the Human Oncology and Pathogenesis Program (HOPP) at Memorial Sloan-Kettering Cancer Center (MSKCC), where he is building a program of lab-based translational researchers across various clinical disciplines and institutional infrastructure to enhance the application of global genomics tools to clinical trials.

Dr. Sawyers' laboratory is currently focused on characterizing signal transduction pathway abnormalities in prostate cancer, with an eye toward translational implications. His research is best demonstrated through his earlier studies of BCR-ABL tyrosine kinase function in chronic myeloid leukemia, his work with Brian Druker and Novartis in the development of the kinase inhibitor imatinib/Gleevec as primary therapy for CML, and his discovery that imatinib resistance is caused by BCR-ABL kinase domain mutations. This discovery led Dr. Sawyers to evaluate second-generation Abl kinase inhibitors, such as the dual Src/Abl inhibitor dasatinib, which received fast-track approval at the FDA in June 2006.

Dr. Sawyers' work in prostate cancer has defined critical signaling pathways for disease initiation and progression through studies in mouse models and humane tissues. This preclinical work led to the development of a novel antiandrogen MVD3100, a small molecule inhibitor discovered in collaboration with UCLA Chemist Michael Jung, which targets the increased levels of androgen receptor found in the hormone refractory disease. Based on impressive clinical results in a phase I/II study, MDV3100 is currently in phase III registration trial. Dr. Sawyers is past President of the American Society of Clinical Investigation and served on the National Cancer Institute's Board of Scientific Councilors. He has won numerous honors and awards, including the Richard and Hinda Rosenthal Foundation Award; the Dorothy Landon Prize from the American Association of Cancer Research; the David A. Karnofsky Award from the American Society of Clinical Oncology; and the 2009 Lasker DeBakey Clinical Medical Research Award. He is a member of the Institute of Medicine and in 2010 was elected to the National Academy of Sciences.

David R. Cox, M.D., Ph.D., serves as Chief Scientific Officer for the Applied Quantitative Genotherapeutics Unit of Pfizer's Worldwide Research & Development. This new unit brings together human genetics, systems biology, and cell biology, combining internal capabilities with outside collaborations, to focus on increasing preclinical target validation with the aim of significantly improving clinical survival. Dr. Cox is a co-founder of Perlegen, and was most recently Chief Scientific Officer of the company since its formation in 2000. Dr. Cox was Professor of Genetics and Pediatrics at the Stanford University School of Medicine as well as the co-director of the Stanford Genome Center. He obtained his A.B. and M.S. degrees from Brown University and his M.D. and Ph.D. degrees from the University of Washington, Seattle. He completed a pediatric residency at the Yale-New Haven Hospital and was a Fellow in both genetics and pediatrics at the University of California, San Francisco. Dr. Cox is certified by the American Board of Pediatrics and the American Board of Medical Genetics. He was an active participant in the large-scale mapping and sequencing efforts of the Human Genome Project while carrying out research involving the molecular basis of human genetic disease. Dr. Cox has been a member of several commissions and boards, including the National Bioethics Advisory Commission (NBAC) and the Health Sciences Policy Board of the Institute of Medicine. He has also served on a number of international committees, including the Council of the Human Genome Organization (HUGO). He has authored over 100 peer-reviewed scientific publications and has served on numerous editorial boards. Dr. Cox's honors include election to the Institute of Medicine of the National Academy of Sciences.

Claire M. Fraser-Liggett is Director of the Institute for Genome Sciences and a Professor of Medicine at the University of Maryland School of Medicine in Baltimore. Previously she was the President and Director of the Institute for Genomic Research in Rockville, Maryland. Dr. Fraser-Liggett has played a role in the sequencing and analysis of human, animal, plant and microbial genomes to better understand the role that genes play in development, evolution, physiology, and disease. She led the teams that sequenced the genomes of several microbial organisms, including important human and animal pathogens, and as a consequence helped to initiate the era of comparative genomics. She has served on a number of National Research Council Committees on counterbioterrorism, domestic animal genomics, polar biology, and metagenomics. Dr. Fraser-Liggett has more than 220 scientific publications, and has served on committees of the National Science Foundation, Department of Energy, and National Institutes of Health. She received her Ph.D. in pharmacology from the State University of New York at Buffalo.

Stephen J. Galli received his B.A. and M.D. from Harvard, in 1968 and 1973, respectively, and completed a residency and chief residency in Anatomic Pathology at Massachusetts General Hospital (MGH) in 1977. After postdoctoral work with Harold F. Dvorak at MGH, he served on the faculty at Harvard Medical School from 1979 until 1999, when he moved to Stanford as Chair of the Department of Pathology, Chief of Pathology at Stanford Hospital & Clinics, Professor of Pathology and of Microbiology and Immunology, and the Mary Hewitt Loveless, MD Professor. He is also Co-Director of the Stanford Center for Genomics and Personalized Medicine. Dr. Galli's research focuses on the development and function of mast cells and basophils (key players in anaphylaxis, allergies, asthma and many other biological responses), and on developing new animal models to study the diverse roles of these cells in health and disease. Dr. Galli serves on the editorial boards of several medical journals and is a co-editor of the *Annual Review of Pathology: Mechanisms of Disease*. He received a MERIT Award from the National Institutes of Health (1995), Scientific Achievement Awards from the International Association of Allergy & Clinical Immunology (1997), and the World Allergy Organization (2011), and is an Honorary Fellow of the College of American Pathologists. He was President of the American Society for Investigative Pathology (2005–2006) and has been elected to the Pluto Club (Association of University Pathologists), the Collegium Internationale Allergologicum (he began a four year term as President in 2010), the American Society for Clinical Investigation, the Association of American Physicians, the Institute of Medicine of the National Academies, and the Accademia Nazionale dei Lincei (the National Academy of the Lynxes) in Rome, considered the oldest secular scientific society in the Western world. In 2006–2007, the last year of a three-year elected term, Dr. Galli was the Chair of the Advisory Board to the President and Provost of Stanford University.

David B. Goldstein is currently Professor of Molecular Genetics & Microbiology and Director of the Center for Human Genome Variation at Duke University. He received his Ph.D. in Biological Sciences from Stanford University in 1994, and from 1999 to 2005 was Wolfson Professor of Genetics at University College London. Dr. Goldstein is the author of over 150 scholarly publications in the areas of population and medical genetics. His work focuses on the genetics of human disease and treatment response, with a concentration on neuropsychiatric disease and host determinants of response to infectious diseases. He is the recipient of one of the first seven nationally awarded Royal Society/Wolfson research merit awards in the UK for his work in human population genetics and was awarded the *Triangle Business Journal* Health Care Heroes Award in 2008 for his work on host determinants of control of HIV-1. Most recently, he was appointed the Co-Chair and Chair of the Gordon Research Conference meeting on human genetics and genomics for 2011 and 2013.

David J. Hunter is currently the Dean for Academic Affairs at the Harvard School of Public Health and the Vincent L. Gregory Professor in Cancer Prevention in the Departments of Epidemiology and Nutrition. His research interests include cancer epidemiology and molecular and genetic epidemiology. Dr. Hunter analyzes inherited susceptibility to cancer and other chronic diseases using molecular techniques and studying molecular markers of environmental exposures. He is Co-Chair of the NCI Breast and Prostate Cancer Cohort Consortium and Co-Director of the NCI Cancer Genetic Markers of Susceptibility (CGEMS) Special Initiative.

Isaac (Zak) S. Kohane is Director of the Children's Hospital Informatics Program and is the Henderson Professor of Pediatrics and Health Sciences and Technology at Harvard Medical School (HMS). He is also Co-Director of the HMS Center for Biomedical Informatics and Director of the HMS Countway Library of Medicine. Dr. Kohane leads multiple collaborations at Harvard Medical School and its hospital affiliates in the use of genomics and computer science to study diseases (particularly cancer and autism). He has developed several computer systems to allow multiple hospital systems to be used as "living laboratories" to study the genetic basis of disease while preserving patient privacy. Among these, the i2b2 (Informatics for Integrating Biology and the Bedside) National Computing Center has been deployed at over 52 academic health centers internationally.

Dr. Kohane has published over 180 papers in the medical literature and authored a widely used book on microarrays for integrative genomics. He has been elected to multiple honor societies including the American Society for Clinical Investigation, the American College of Medical Informatics, and the Institute of Medicine. He leads a doctoral program in genomics and bioinformatics at the Division of Health Sciences and Technology at Harvard and MIT. He is also a practicing pediatrics endocrinologist and father of three energetic children.

Manuel Llinás is an Assistant Professor of Molecular Biology and a member of the Lewis-Sigler Institute for Integrative Genomics at Princeton University. Dr. Llinás earned a Ph.D. in molecular and cell biology from the University of California-Berkeley and did postdoctoral work in the lab of Joseph DeRisi at the University of California-San Francisco. He joined the Princeton faculty in 2005. Dr. Llinás' laboratory studies the deadliest of the four human Plasmodium parasites, *Plasmodium falciparum*. His research combines tools from functional genomics, molecular biology, computational biology, biochemistry, and metabolomics to understand the fundamental molecular mechanisms underlying the development of this parasite. The focus is predominantly on the red blood cell stage of development, which is the stage in which all of the clinical manifestations of the malaria disease occur. His research has focused on two major areas: the role of transcriptional regulation in orchestrating parasite development, and an in-depth characterization of the malaria parasite's unique metabolic network. On the transcription side, Dr. Llinás' lab works on the characterization of the first family of DNA binding proteins to be identified in the *P. falciparum* genome, the Apicomplexan AP2 (ApiAP2) proteins. The metabolomics work has begun to identify unique biochemical pathway architectures in the parasite including a novel branched TCA cycle. These two approaches explore relatively virgin areas in the malaria field with the goal of identifying novel strategies for therapeutic intervention.

Bernard Lo, M.D., is Professor of Medicine and Director of the Program in Medical Ethics at UCSF. He is also National Program Director for the Greenwall Faculty Scholars Program in Bioethics, a career development award for bioethics researchers. He directs the Regulatory Knowledge Support Component of the NIH-funded Clinical and Translational Science Institute at UCSF and is Co-Director of the Policy and Ethics Core of the Center for AIDS Prevention Studies. He chairs the UCSF Stem Cell Research Oversight Committee. He is Co-Chair of the Standards Working Group of the California Institute of Regenerative Medicine, which recommends regulations for stem cell research funded by the state of California. He is a member of the Centers for Disease Control and Prevention (CDC) Ethics Subcommittee of the Advisory Committee to the Director. He serves on DSMBs for NIH-sponsored HIV vaccine trials, the Long-Term Oxygen Treatment Trial (LOTT), and on the Ethics Working Group of the HIV Prevention Trials Network. He also serves on the Board of Directors of the Association for the Accreditation of Human Research Protection Programs. He is a member of the Institute of Medicine (IOM), served on the IOM Council and as chair of the IOM Board on Health Sciences Policy. He chaired a 2009 IOM Committee on conflicts of interest in medicine and several earlier reports. Dr. Lo is author of *Resolving Ethical Dilemmas: A Guide for Clinicians* (4th ed., 2010) and of *Ethical Issues in Clinical Research* (2010).

Tom Misteli is a Senior Investigator and Head of the Cell Biology of Genomes group at the National Cancer Institute, NIH. Dr. Misteli obtained his Ph.D. from the University of London, UK, and joined the NCI after postdoctoral work at the Cold Spring Harbor Laboratory, New York. He has pioneered the field of genome cell biology by developing live-cell microscopy approaches to study the nuclear organization of the genome and gene expression in intact cells, and his laboratory aims to apply this knowledge to the development of novel diagnostic and therapeutic strategies for cancer and aging. Dr. Misteli has received numerous awards for his work, and currently serves as Editor-in-Chief of the *Journal of Cell Biology* and of *Current Opinion in Cell Biology*.

Sean J. Morrison, Ph.D., is the Director of the Children's Research Institute and the Mary McDermott Cook Chair in Pediatric Genetics at the University of Texas Southwestern Medical Center as well as an Investigator of the Howard Hughes Medical Institute.

The Morrison laboratory is investigating the mechanisms that regulate stem cell function in the nervous and hematopoietic systems and the ways in which these mechanisms are hijacked by cancer cells to enable neoplastic proliferation and metastasis. The Morrison laboratory is particularly interested in the mechanisms that regulate stem cell self-renewal, stem cell aging, and the role these mechanisms play in cancer. Parallel studies of these mechanisms in two tissues reveals the extent to which different types of stem cells and cancer cells depend upon similar mechanisms to regulate their function.

The Morrison laboratory has discovered a number of critical mechanisms that distinguish stem cell self-renewal from the proliferation of restricted progenitors. They have shown that stem cell self-renewal is regulated by networks of proto-oncogenes and tumor suppressors and that the balance between proto-oncogenic and tumor suppressor signals changes with age. This likely explains why the mutation spectrum changes with age in cancer patients, as different mechanisms become competent to hyper-activate self-renewal pathways in patients at different ages. The Morrison laboratory has further shown that in some cancers many tumor cells are capable of driving disease growth and progression while other cancers are driven by minority subpopulations of cancer cells that adopt "stem cell" characteristics. These insights into the cellular and molecular mechanisms of self-renewal have suggested new approaches for promoting normal tissue regeneration and cancer treatment.

Dr. Morrison completed a BSc in biology and chemistry at Dalhousie University (1991), then a Ph.D. in immunology at Stanford University (1996), and a postdoctoral fellowship in neurobiology at the California Institute of Technology (Caltech; 1999). From 1999 to 2011, Dr. Morrison was at the University of Michigan where he directed the Center for Stem Cell Biology. Recently, Dr. Morrison moved to the University of Texas Southwestern Medical Center where he is the founding Director of the new Children's Research Institute. Dr. Morrison was a Searle Scholar (2000–2003), received the Presidential Early Career Award for Scientists and Engineers (2003), the International Society for Hematology and Stem Cell's McCulloch and Till Award (2007), the American

Association of Anatomists Harland Mossman Award (2008), and a MERIT Award from the National Institute on Aging (2009).

Dr. Morrison has also been active in public policy issues surrounding stem cell research. For example, he has twice testified before Congress and was a leader in the successful "Proposal 2" campaign to protect stem cell research in Michigan's state constitution.

David G. Nichols is Professor of Anesthesiology/Critical Care Medicine and Pediatrics and the Mary Wallace Stanton Professor of Education at Johns Hopkins University. Since joining the School of Medicine faculty in 1984, he has held numerous leadership posts in both the Department of Anesthesiology and Critical Care Medicine and school-wide. Named Vice Dean for Education in 2000, Dr. Nichols oversees undergraduate, graduate, residency, postdoctoral and continuing medical education programs, as well as the Welch Medical Library. He has led a wide variety of significant initiatives to improve the School of Medicine's innovative use of technology in education; update the Medical School's curriculum; improve faculty development by revising tenure and promotion guidelines; restructure graduate medical education; oversee the design of a new $50 million medical education building; and enhance diversity throughout Johns Hopkins Medicine.

From 1984 to 1987, Dr. Nichols was Associate Director of the Residency Education Program in the Department of Anesthesiology and Critical Care Medicine. He became Director of the Division of Pediatric Critical Care and of the pediatric intensive care unit (PICU) in 1988. The division was merged with pediatric anesthesiology under Dr. Nichols' leadership in 1997. During this period, he trained and mentored more than 50 postdoctoral fellows, many of whom now are professors or directors of PICUs in the United States and abroad. Dr. Nichols became a full professor of anesthesiology/critical care medicine and pediatrics in 1998 and became the recipient of the Mary Wallace Stanton Professorship for Education in 2005. He has written more than 80 professional journal articles and abstracts, held 17 guest professorships, headed more than 20 symposia, and delivered more than 115 guest lectures. He also has been editor-in-chief of the leading textbooks in pediatric critical care medicine and edited *Rogers Textbook of Pediatric Intensive Care* and *Critical Heart Disease in Infants and Children*.

Maynard V. Olson is Professor Emeritus of Medicine and Genome Sciences at the University of Washington. He received his Ph.D. in Chemistry at Stanford University in 1970 and a BS in Chemistry from the California Institute of Technology in 1965. His research interests focus on studies of natural genetic variation in both bacteria and humans. This research involves activities in human genetics, genomics, molecular genetics, analytical biochemistry, and computational biology. Dr. Olson has a special interest in interdisciplinary research, particularly at the interfaces between chemistry, computer science, and biology.

Dr. Olson was involved in shaping scientific policy toward the Human Genome Project, serving on the National Research Council Committee on Mapping and Sequencing the Human Genome, the Program Advisory Committee of the National Center for Human Genome Research Institute. In recognition of his research in genetics and genomics, he received the Genetics Society of America Medal in 1992, the City of Medicine Award in 2000, the Gairdner International Award in 2002, and the Gruber Prize in Genetics in 2007.

Charmaine D. Royal is an Associate Research Professor in the Institute for Genome Sciences & Policy and the Department of African and African American Studies at Duke University. She received her M.S. in Genetic Counseling and Ph.D. in Human Genetics from Howard University. She subsequently completed her postdoctoral training in the Bioethics and Special Populations Research Program at the National Human Genome Research Institute of the National Institutes of Health, and in the Division of Epidemiology and Behavioral Medicine at the Howard University Cancer Center.

Prior to joining the Duke faculty in 2007, Dr. Royal was Assistant Professor of Pediatrics and Director of the GenEthics Unit in the National Human Genome Center at Howard University. She serves on the Bioethics Advisory Committee of the March of Dimes Foundation, Social Issues Committee of the American Society of Human Genetics, Editorial Board of the *American Journal of Bioethics*, and various other professional committees and boards.

Dr. Royal's research and scholarship focus primarily on ethical, psychosocial, societal, and biomedical issues at the intersection of genetics/genomics and concepts of "race", ancestry, ethnicity, and identity. Her specific interests include genetic variation and the (re)conceptualization of race, use of race and ancestry in research and clinical practice, gene-environment interactions in health and health disparities, genetic ancestry inference, involvement of historically marginalized and underrepresented groups in genetic and genomic research, and genomics and global health. She has taught, presented, published, and received funding in these and other related areas. A key objective of her research program is to advance a more holistic and ethical approach to understanding and improving human health and well-being through increased integration of genetic and genomic research with behavioral, social science, and humanities research.

Keith R. Yamamoto, Ph.D., is Professor of Cellular and Molecular Pharmacology and Executive Vice Dean of the School of Medicine at the University of California, San Francisco. He has been a member of the UCSF faculty since 1976, serving as Director of the PIBS Graduate Program in Biochemistry and Molecular Biology (1988–2003), Vice Chair of the Department of Biochemistry and Biophysics (1985–1994), Chair of the Department of Cellular and Molecular Pharmacology (1994–2003), and Vice Dean for Research, School of Medicine (2002–2003). Dr. Yamamoto's research is focused on signaling and transcriptional regulation by intracellular receptors, which mediate the actions of several classes of essential hormones and cellular signals; he uses both mechanistic and systems approaches to pursue these problems in pure molecules, cells, and whole organisms. Dr. Yamamoto was a founding editor of *Molecular Biology of the Cell*, and serves on numerous editorial boards and scientific advisory boards, and national committees focused on public and scientific policy, public understanding and support of biological research, and science education; he chairs the Coalition for the Life Sciences (formerly the Joint Steering Committee for Public Policy) and for the National Academy of Sciences, he chairs the Board on Life Sciences. Dr. Yamamoto has long been involved in the process of peer review and the policies that govern it at the National Institutes of Health, serving as Chair of the Molecular Biology Study Section, member of the NIH Director's Working Group on the Division of Research Grants, Chair of the Advisory Committee to the NIH Center for Scientific Review (CSR), member of the NIH Director's Peer Review Oversight Group, member of the CSR Panel on Scientific Boundaries for Review, member of the Advisory Committee to the NIH Director, Co-Chair of the Working Group to Enhance NIH Peer Review, and Co-Chair of the Review Committee for the Transformational R01 Award. Dr. Yamamoto was elected as a member of the American Academy of Arts and Sciences in 1988, the National Academy of Sciences in 1989, the Institute of Medicine in 2003, and as a fellow of the American Association for the Advancement of Sciences in 2002.

NATIONAL RESEARCH COUNCIL STAFF

India Hook-Barnard is a program officer with the Board on Life Sciences of the National Research Council. She came to the National Academies from the National Institutes of Health where she was a Postdoctoral Research Fellow from 2003 to 2008. Her research investigating the molecular mechanism of gene expression focused on the interactions between RNA polymerase and promoter DNA. Dr. Hook-Barnard earned her Ph.D. from the Department of Molecular Microbiology and Immunology at the University of Missouri. Her graduate research examined translational regulation and ribosome binding in *Escherichia coli*. At the National Academies, she contributes to projects in a variety of topic areas. Much of her current work is related to issues of molecular biology, microbiology, biosecurity, and genomics. She was study director for the 2010 report *Sequence-Based Classification of Select Agents: A Brighter Line,* and continues to direct the U.S. National Committee to the International Brain Research Organization.

Orin Luke is a Program Assistant with the Board on Life Sciences of the National Research Council. He received a B.A. in English from the University of Maryland, College Park. Since joining the Board on Life Sciences in 2011, he has served as Program Assistant for a variety of projects, including *Molecular Dynamics* (2011), *Evolution Across the Curriculum* (2011), and *Continuing Assistance to the National Institutes of Health on Preparation of Additional Risk Assessments for the Boston University NEIDL* (2011) among others. Prior to joining the Board on Life Sciences he was a Program Assistant with the Board on Environmental Studies and Toxicology.

Amanda Mazzawi most recently worked at The National Academy of the Sciences as a Senior Program Assistant, where she had the opportunity to assist in the logistical planning and implantation of multiple meetings, projects, documents and reports. Prior to her work at NAS she spent two years working closely with senior management at the North Carolina State University's Center for Excellence in Curricular Engagement. She lead projects and implemented programs that have greatly expanded student participation in student/community involvement programs across the NCSU campus and surrounding communities to facilitate the concept of Service-Learning. Amanda currently lives in Ithaca, NY with her husband and 2 month old son.

Carl-Gustav Anderson is a Program Associate with the Board on Life Sciences of the National Research Council. He received a B.A. in Philosophy from American University in 2009. He is currently completing his M.A. in the History of Philosophy at American University. Before joined the Board on Life Sciences in 2009, he worked closely with the All Women's Action Society (Malaysia), helping to engage young men in feminist dialogue and to present a feminist response to the unique identity politics of contemporary Malaysia. His current research focuses on the potential contributions of Buddhist philosophy and American pragmatism to feminist and queer epistemologies.

Since joining the Board on Life Sciences in 2009, he has served as Program Associate for variety of projects, including *Responsible Research with Biological Select Agents and Toxins* (2009), *Challenges and Opportunities for Education about Dual Use Issues in Life Sciences Research* (2010), *Sequence-Based Classification of Select Agents: A Brighter Line* (2010), *Evaluation of a Site-Specific Risk Assessment for the Department of Homeland Security's Planned National Bio- and Agro-Defense Facility in Manhattan, Kansas* (2010), *Challenges and Opportunities for Education About Dual Use Issues in the Life Sciences* (2010), *Protecting the Frontline in Biodefense Research: The Special Immunizations Program* (2011), and *Research in the Life Sciences with Dual Use Potential: An International Faculty Development Project on Education About the Responsible Conduct of Science* (2011), among others. In addition to several ongoing studies, he also serves as Program Associate for the United States-Canada Regional Committee to the International Brain Research Organization.

Appendix C

March 1& 2, 2011—Workshop Agenda

Framework for Developing a New Taxonomy of Disease

Tuesday and Wednesday, March 1 and 2, 2011
The House of Sweden—Alfred Nobel Hall
Washington, DC

AGENDA
Day 1

Breakfast available at 7:15 am in the Atrium Lounge

8:00 AM **SESSION 1: WELCOME AND OPENING TALKS**
- **Committee co-chairs:**
  o **Susan Desmond-Hellmann:** *Chancellor, UCSF*
  o **Charles Sawyers:** *Director of HOPP, Memorial Sloan-Kettering Cancer Center*
- **Chris Chute:** *Professor of Medical Informatics, Mayo Clinic College of Medicine*—Current Taxonomy: importance, process of updating ICD
- **Atul Butte:** *Chief and Assistant Professor, Division of Systems Medicine, Department of Pediatrics, Stanford*—Current Taxonomy transitioning to New Taxonomy

9:20 AM **Break**

9:35 AM **A NEW TAXONOMY NETWORK—Keith Yamamoto** A proposal for consideration and further development.

10:00 AM **SESSION 2: DO WE NEED AN AMERICAN GENOMES PROJECT?**
A panel discussion—David Goldstein, Moderator
Is genomic information central to a New Taxonomy of Disease? What are the opportunities and concerns? What is

happening now with whole-genome sequencing? What are the goals in near/ long term?—Define productive pathways.
Andrew Conrad: *Chief Scientific Officer, LabCorp's NGI*
Kathy Giusti: *Founder and Chief Executive Officer, Multiple Myeloma Research Foundation (MMRF)*

Panel discussion: ~30 min

11:00 AM **SESSION 3: BEYOND THE GENOME—INFORMATION FOR A NEW TAXONOMY**
A panel discussion—Manuel Llinas, Moderator
In addition to genome sequence, other information could be leveraged to improve health and research as part of a New Taxonomy of Disease Network. What information could/ should be included in the network? Would this enable longitudinal studies?
Lewis Cantley: *Chief, Division of Signal Transduction, Harvard Medical School*—Metabolome, proteome
Martin Blaser: —*Frederick H. King Professor of Internal Medicine and Chairman of the Department of Medicine, NYU School of Medicine*—Microbiome
Jason Lieb: *Professor, Department of Biology, UNC*—Epigenetics; ENCODE project
Helmut Zarbl: *UMDNJ-Robert Wood Johnson Medical School, Environmental & Occupational Medicine, Rutgers University*—Environmental Health, toxicology
Erin Ramos: *Epidemiologist, National Human Genome Research Institute*—Sociological contributions, PhenX

Panel discussion: ~30 min

12:45 PM **Lunch**

1:30 PM **SESSION 4: ETHICS AND PRIVACY**
A panel discussion—Bernie Lo, Moderator
Alta Charo: *Professor of Law and Bioethics, University of Wisconsin Law School*—Informed Consent, Privacy
Sanford Schwartz: *Professor of Medicine, Health Care Management, and Economics, University of Pennsylvania*—Clinical validation issues
Debra Lappin: *President, Council for American Medical Innovation*—Patient Advocate

Panel discussion: ~30 min

3:00 PM   **Break**

3:30 PM   **SESSION 5: PRODUCT DEVELOPMENT—PHARMA;
            BIOTECH**
            A panel discussion—David Cox; Moderator
            1. How would a New Taxonomy of human disease enable
               more cost-effective and rapid development of new, effective,
               and safe drugs in the pharma/biotech setting?
            2. How would a New Taxonomy of human disease promote
               integration of clinical and research cultures in the pharma/
               biotech industry?
            3. How would a New Taxonomy of human disease promote
               public/private partnerships between industry and academia?
            4. What are key factors that would limit the implementation of
               a New Taxonomy of human disease in the pharma/biotech
               setting?
            • **Klaus Lindpaintner:** *Vice President of R&D, SDI*
            • **Charles Baum:** *Vice President of Global R&D, Pfizer*
            • **Corey Goodman:** *Managing Director and Co-Founder,
              venBio*

            Panel discussion: ~30 min

5:00 PM   **Summary of the day, overview of tomorrow, discussion: Susan
            Desmond-Hellmann and Charles Sawyers**

AGENDA
Day 2

Breakfast available at 7:15 am in the Atrium Lounge

8:00 AM   **Opening Remarks: Susan Desmond-Hellmann and Charles
            Sawyers**

8:10 AM   **SESSION 6: PRAGMATIC CONSIDERATIONS—
            THE END USER**
            **A panel discussion—David Hunter and David Nichols;
            Moderators**
            1. What taxonomy framework would be most useful for your
               end-user group? Why?

2. What characteristics of a taxonomy framework might harm your end-user group? Why?
3. What criteria should be used to assess the value of a New Taxonomy? (cost, ethics, practicality, health-care outcomes, etc.?)
4. Should the lay public be able to comprehend a New Taxonomy of Disease?

- **Janet Woodcock:** *Director, CDER/FDA*
- **Jon Lorsch:** *Professor of Biophysics and Biophysical Chemistry, Johns Hopkins University, School of Medicine*
- **Brian Kelly:** *Head of Informatics and Strategic Alignment, Aetna*
- **Sanford Schwartz:** *Professor of Medicine, Health Care Management, and Economics, University of Pennsylvania—* Cost Effectiveness Issues

Panel discussion: ~30 min

10:00 AM   **Break**

10:15 AM   **SESSION 7: INSTRUMENTING THE HEALTH CARE DELIVERY SYSTEM TO DEFINE AND LEVERAGE A NEW TAXONOMY**
A panel discussion—Isaac Kohane, Moderator
Considerations for cognition, data handling, visualization and user interface.

- **Daniel Masys:** *Chair of the Department of Biomedical Informatics, Vanderbilt University Medical Center—* eMERGE consortium (using health care data to run genomic studies)
- **John Brownstein:** *Instructor, Harvard Medical School—* Informal data sources,Health map.org

Panel discussion: ~30 min

12:00 PM   **Lunch**

12:45 PM   **SESSION 8: A CLINICAL PERSPECTIVE ON A NEW TAXONOMY Case Studies—Charles Sawyers, Moderator**
Physician/Scientists consider what a New Taxonomy of Disease would mean for the disease they study.

- **William Pao:** *Director, Personalized Cancer Medicine at the Vanderbilt-Ingram Cancer Center—*Lung Cancer

- **Ingrid Scheffer:** *Professor of Paediatric Neurology Research, University of Melbourne*—Epilepsy
- **Elissa Epel:** *Associate Professor in Residence, Department of Psychiatry at UCSF*—Chronic Stress/ Obesity

Panel discussion: ~30 min

2:15 PM   **Final discussion and Closing Remarks: Susan Desmond-Hellmann and Charles Sawyers**
(Committee will meet for an hour in closed session)

3:00 PM   **Adjourn**

Appendix D

eMERGE Consortium
Data Use Agreement

Data Use Agreement

For use by and among
Members of the Electronic Medical Records and Genomics Research
Network (eMERGE)

TERMS AND DEFINITIONS: The Electronic Medical Records and Genomics (eMERGE) Network (https://www.mc.vanderbilt.edu/victr/dcc/projects/acc/index.php/About) is a National Institutes of Health (NIH)-organized and -funded consortium of U.S. medical research institutions ("eMERGE Network"). The primary goal of the eMERGE Network is to develop, disseminate, and apply approaches to research that combine DNA biorepositories with electronic medical record (EMR) systems for large-scale, high-throughput genetic research. Member institutions participating in the consortium study the relationship between genetic variations and clinically relevant human traits, using the technique of genome-wide association (GWAS) analysis. Such studies involve testing hundreds of thousands of genetic variants called single nucleotide polymorphisms throughout the genome in people with and without a condition of interest. A fundamental question that eMERGE seeks to answer is whether electronic medical record (EMR) systems can serve as resources for such complex genomic analysis of disease susceptibility and therapeutic outcomes, across diverse patient populations. In addition, the consortium includes a focus on social and ethical issues such as privacy, confidentiality, and interactions with the broader community. Detailed information on the eMERGE network can be found at the eMERGE website (www.gwas.org).

The following entities are eMERGE Network members ("eMERGE Network Members" or "Members"): Group Health/University of Washington, Marshfield Clinic, Mayo Clinic, Northwestern University and Vanderbilt University serve as the clinical sites ("Clinical Sites"); Vanderbilt University also serves as the consortium's coordinating center ("Coordinating Center"); Broad Institute and Center for Inherited Disease Research both serve as genotyping facilities ("Genotyping Facilities"); and the National Center for Biotechnology Information (NCBI), NIH; and the National Human Genome Research Institute (NHGRI), NIH ("Program Officials") serve as scientific and programmatic managers and technical advisors.

Researchers with a wide range of expertise in genomics, statistics, ethics, informatics, and clinical medicine employed by an eMERGE Network Member participate in the eMERGE network, including: Principal Investigators of the eMERGE Clinical Sites, the Coordinating Center, the Genotyping Facilities, and Program Officials from the National Center for Biotechnology Information and the National Human Genome Research Institute.

Data Sharing Guiding Principles: All data sharing will adhere to 1) the terms of consent agreed to by research participants; 2) applicable laws and regulations, and; 3) the principle that individual sites within the network have final authority regarding whether their site's data will be used or shared, on a per-project basis. These principles are intended to maximize sharing of GWAS data generated by the eMERGE Members among and between other Members as well as with the wider scientific community, and to do this without compromising data security or the confidentiality of information about individuals whose data and/or samples are used for research.

Data Sharing Responsibilities: Principal Investigators of each eMERGE Clinical Site may designate data to accomplish activities defined in eMERGE sanctioned research studies (eMERGE data) to be shared as follows: (1) distribution through dbGaP; (2) distribution within the eMERGE Network; and/or (3) distribution to the eMERGE Coordinating Center. The eMERGE data to be shared within eMERGE will be provided only to eMERGE Network Members that have signed this Agreement. All eMERGE Network Members and the eMERGE Coordinating Center may aggregate eMERGE data from all Member sites and, with documented approval prior to each submission from the contributing site(s), submit said eMERGE data to dbGaP and/or other databases administered by the National Institutes of Health. Each eMERGE Network Member may share its own data with external collaborators without approval of the other Members. If eMERGE data received from any Member is shared externally by another Member, prior approval from the Member providing the eMERGE data must be obtained and documented. Members sharing eMERGE data externally must also ensure that each external eMERGE data recipient agrees to the same restrictions and conditions applicable to Members and Member Representatives regarding the use and disclosure of the eMERGE data as outlined in this Agreement or as may be required by law.

Statement of Confidentiality: By signing this Agreement, the authorized official representing an eMERGE Network Member, certifies that s/he and the Principal Investigators, fellows, students, and research staff (collectively, "Network Member Representatives") working on eMERGE-related projects are aware of the confidential nature of data on research participants maintained by the Member and of the necessity for maintaining that confidentiality.

The eMERGE Network Member agrees not to attempt to personally identify any eMERGE participant based on eMERGE data and agree not to attempt to contact any eMERGE participant of a site other than their own. The Member agrees not to transfer or disclose any confidential data or any information about individual eMERGE participants, except as permitted by this Agreement or as required by law, either during or after the conclusion of the affiliation with eMERGE. The Member agrees to provide adequate security for the eMERGE data, including but not limited to safeguards intended to prevent unauthorized use or disclosure of such information. In addition each Member agrees to report in writing to the other Members any use or disclosure of any portion of the data of which it becomes aware that is not permitted by this Agreement including disclosures that are required by law.

The eMERGE Network Member agrees to ensure that its Network Member Representatives do not use, disclose or transfer any eMERGE data to anyone who is not an eMERGE Network Member except as permitted by this Agreement or as required by law. Further, the Member agrees to return all eMERGE data to the eMERGE Coordinating Center or delete/destroy all electronic eMERGE data upon termination of its affiliation with the eMERGE Network and to notify the eMERGE Coordinating Center when it has done so.

Limitations of Data Use: The eMERGE Network Member agrees to ensure that Network Member Representatives will only use eMERGE data in a manner that is consistent with any limitations that have been specified for individual studies by the disclosing Member and agreed to by the Steering Committee and shall ensure compliance with all applicable state and federal laws and regulations governing the use of such data including the Health Insurance Portability and Accountability Act of 1996 (HIPAA), if applicable, including any and all future amendments.

The eMERGE Network Member agrees to comply with all established policies of eMERGE governing the acquisition, analysis, reporting, publication, use and distribution of eMERGE data.

This Agreement supersedes and replaces all prior agreements made between eMERGE Network Members.

Agreed to by:

eMERGE Institution Authorized Official name and title (print): _____
Signature: _____   Date: _____

Read & Understood by:
Network Member Representative name & title (print): _____
Signature: _____   Date: _____
Member Representative's Institution:
_____

Appendix E

Glossary

Biobank a bank of biological specimens for biomedical research.

Biomarker a characteristic that is objectively measured and evaluated as an indicator of normal biological processes, pathogenic processes, or pharmacologic responses to a therapeutic intervention (IOM 2010a).

Biosamples Samples of biological materials

Candidate gene a gene whose chromosomal location is associated with a particular disease or other phenotype. Because of its location, the gene is suspected of causing the disease or other phenotype (NHGRI 2011).

Chromosomal translocation a condition where a fragment of one chromosome is broken off and is then attached to another. Depending on which piece of chromosome is moved to where, this results in a wide range of medical problems, such as leukemia, breast cancer, schizophrenia, or muscular dystrophy (USC 2011).

Clinical utility the ability of a screening or diagnostic test to prevent or ameliorate adverse health outcomes such as mortality, morbidity, or disability through the adoption of efficacious treatments conditioned on test results (Khoury 2003).

Crowd sourcing informal reports of large groups of people

Database of Genotypes and Phenotypes (dbGap) developed to archive and distribute the results of studies that have investigated the interaction of genotype and phenotype (NCBI 2011).

Data-intensive biology understanding of biological processes through models and algorithms of mathematics, statistics, and computer science using the vast volumes of data generated by new technologies (http://sc11.supercomputing. org/schedule/event_detail.php?evid=wksp120).

Decision-support systems a specific class of computerized information system that supports business and organizational decision-making activities (Information Builders 2011).

Disease marker specific molecular signature of disease, physiological measurement, genotype structural or functional characteristic, metabolic changes, or other determinant that may simplify the diagnostic process, make diagnoses more accurate, distinguish different causes of disease, or enable physicians to make diagnoses before symptoms appear and to track disease progression (Medical Dictionary 2011)

Disease risk the probability that an individual who is initially disease-free will developed given disease over specified time or age interval (e.g. one year or lifetime) (Pigeot 2005).

Disease taxonomy the science of disease classification.

DNA (Deoxyribonucleic acid) the polymer that encodes genetic material and therefore the structures of proteins and many animal traits.

EHR (Electronic Health Record) a subset of each CDO's EMR, presently assumed to include summaries, such as ASTM's Continuity of Care Record (CCR) and HL7's Care Record Summary (CRS), and possibly information from pharmacy benefit management firms, reference labs and other organizations about the health status of patients in the community (Garets and Davis 2005).

EHR-derived phenotype phenotype based on Electronic Health Record (EHR).

Electronic medical records (EMS) computerized legal clinical records created in CDOs, such as hospitals and physician offices (Garets and Davis 2005).

Epigenetic relating to, being, or involving a modification in gene expression that is independent of the DNA sequence of a gene (e.g., epigenetic carcinogenesis, epigenetic inheritance) (Merriam-Webster 2007).

Epigenome the epigenome consists of chemical compounds that modify, or mark, the genome in a way that tells it what to do, where to do it, and when to do it. Different cells have different epigenetic marks. These epigenetic marks, which are not part of the DNA itself, can be passed on from cell to cell as cells divide, and from one generation to the next (NHGRI 2011).

Epiphenomenon an additional condition or symptom in the course of a disease, not necessarily connected with the disease (Houghton Mifflin Company 2007).

Etiology the study of all factors that may be involved in the development of a disease, including the susceptibility of the patient, the nature of the disease agent, and the way in which the patient's body is invaded by the agent (Mosby 2009).

Exposome characterization of both exogenous and endogenous exposures that can have differential effects at various stages during a person's lifetime (Wild 2005; Rappaport 2011).

Gel electrophoresis electrophoresis in which molecules (as proteins and nucleic acids) migrate through a gel and especially a polyacrylamide gel and separate into bands according to size (Merriam-Webster 2007).

GenBank the GenBank sequence database is an annotated collection of all publicly available nucleotide sequences and their protein translations (Mizrachi 2002).

Gene-environment interactions an influence on the expression of a trait that results from the interplay between genes and the environment. Some traits are strongly influenced by genes, while other traits are strongly influenced by the environment. Most traits, however, are influenced by one or more genes interacting in complex ways with the environment (NHGRI 2011).

Gene expression is the process by which the information encoded in a gene is used to direct the assembly of a protein molecule. The cell reads the sequence of the gene in groups of three bases. Each group of three bases (codon) corresponds to one of 20 different amino acids used to build the protein (NHGRI 2011).

Gene expression profiling is the measurement of the activity of thousands of genes at once to create a global picture of cellular function. These profiles can, for example, distinguish between cells that are actively dividing, or show how the cells react to a particular treatment. Many experiments of this sort measure an entire genome simultaneously, that is, every gene present in a particular cell (InfoGlobalLink 2011).

Genetic polymorphisms the recurrence within a population of two or more discontinuous genetic variants of a specific trait in such proportions that they cannot be maintained simply by mutation. Examples include the sickle cell trait, the Rh factor, and the blood groups (Mosby 2009).

Genetic privacy the protection of genetic information about an individual, family, or population group from unauthorized disclosure (Kahn and Ninomiya 2010).

Genome the full sequence of genetic material encoded in DNA in an organism.

Genome-Wide Association Study (GWAS) a study that identifies markers across genomes to find genetic variation associated with a disease or condition (PCAST 2008).

Genotype the genetic sequence of an individual organism, often categorized in terms of known genetic variants. This can either refer to known alleles (or types) of a single gene or to collections of genes. For example, some lung cancers have a mutant Egf receptor genotype while other lung cancers have a wild-type (or normal) Egf receptor genotype.

Geographic Information System (GIS) an organized collection of computer hardware, software, geographic data, and personnel designed to efficiently capture, store, update, manipulate, analyze, and display all forms of geographically referenced information (ESRI 1990).

Health Insurance Portability and Accountability Act (HIPAA) an act of Congress, passed in 1996, that affords certain protections to persons covered by health-care plans, including continuity of coverage when changing jobs, standards for electronic health-care transactions, and privacy safeguards for individually identifiable patient information (Mosby 2009).

Heterozygous having inherited different forms of a particular gene from each parent. A heterozygous genotype stands in contrast to a homozygous genotype, where an individual inherits identical forms of a particular gene from each parent (NHGRI 2011).

Histology the science dealing with the microscopic identification of cells and tissue (Mosby 2009).

Human Microbiome Project (HMP) a National Institutes of Health initiative that aims to characterize the microbial communities found at several different sites on the human body, including nasal passages, oral cavities, skin, gastrointestinal tract, and urogenital tract, and to analyze the role of these microbes in human health and disease.

Institutional Review Board (IRB) a group of physicians, scientists, ethicists, lawyers, and community members that review human subjects research to ensure that the research will be performed ethically and that it will benefit patients. Individual institutions, such as universities, often have their own IRBs that must approve all human subjects research before it is conducted within the institution.

International Classification of Diseases (ICD) an official list of categories of diseases, physical and mental, issued by the World Health Organization (WHO). It is used primarily for statistical purposes in the classification of morbidity and mortality data. Any nation belonging to WHO may adjust the classification to meet specific needs (Mosby 2009).

Linkage analysis (LA) a gene-hunting technique that traces patterns of heredity in large, high-risk families in an attempt to locate a disease-causing gene mutation by identifying traits co-inherited with it; the formal study of the association between the inheritance of a condition in a family and a particular chromosomal locus; LA is based on certain ground rules of genetics (McGraw-Hill 2002).

Lipidome the totality of lipids in cells (Quehenberger et al. 2010).

Longitudinal study a research study that collects repeated observations of the same items over a long period of time (PCAST 2008).

Metabolic profiling identifying the types and amounts of known metabolic intermediates present in a biological specimen.

Metabolome can be defined as the complete complement of all small molecule (<1500 Da) metabolites found in a specific cell, organ, or organism. It is a close counterpart to the genome, the transcriptome, and the proteome. Together these four 'omes' constitute the building blocks of systems biology (Wishar et al. 2007).

Microbiome term used to describe the collective genome of our indigenous microbed (microflora) (Hooper and Gordon 2001 in IOM 2010b). Identification of the types of microbes present in a biological specimen or that are associated with another organism, such as a human.

Molecular biology (A) a branch of biology dealing with the ultimate physico-chemical organization of living matter and especially with the molecular basis of inheritance and protein synthesis (Merriam-Webster 2007); (B) field of science concerned with the chemical structures and processes of biological phenomena at the molecular level (Merriam-Webster 2007).

Moore's Law the number of transistors that can be placed inexpensively on an integrated circuit doubles approximately every two years (Moore 1965).

National Center for Biotechnology Information (NCBI) the National Center for Biotechnology Information advances science and health by providing access to biomedical and genomic information (NCBI 2011).

Natural language processing a theoretically motivated range of computational techniques for analyzing and representing naturally occurring texts at one or more levels of linguistic analysis for the purpose of achieving human-like language processing for a range of tasks or applications (Liddy 2001)

Observational studies although molecular data will be collected from individuals in the normal course of health care, no changes in the treatment of the individuals would be contingent on the data collected.

Ontology a branch of metaphysics concerned with the nature and relations of being (Merriam-Webster 2007).

Oophorectomy the surgical removal of an ovary (Merriam-Webster 2007).

Outcomes research the systematic study of the effects of different therapeutic interventions on health outcomes.

Pathogenesis the origination and development of a disease (Merriam-Webster 2007).

Pathology (A) the study of the essential nature of diseases and especially of the structural and functional changes produced by them; (B) something abnormal: *a* : the structural and functional deviations from the normal that constitute disease or characterize a particular disease (Merriam-Webster 2007).

Pathophysiology the physiology of abnormal states; *specifically* : the functional changes that accompany a particular syndrome or disease (Merriam-Webster 2007).

Patient oriented research observation and scientific study of individuals or small groups of subjects for an understanding of their physiologic and pathophysiologic characteristics. The primary focus of the research is on mechanisms of disease on the clinical observations and laboratory studies that define these mechanisms as well as interventions that modify the course of the disease (APOR 2011).

Personalized medicine (also see: Precision medicine) "refers to the tailoring of medical treatment to the individual characteristics of each patient. It does not literally mean the creation of drugs or medical devices that are unique to a patient, but rather the ability to classify individuals into subpopulations that differ in their susceptibility to a particular disease or their response to a specific treatment. Preventive or therapeutic interventions can then be concentrated on those who will benefit, sparing expense and side effects for those who will not" (PCAST 2008). This term is now widely used, including in advertisements for commercial products, and it is sometimes misinterpreted as implying that unique treatments can be designed for each individual. For this reason, the Committee thinks that the term "precision medicine" is preferable to "personalized medicine" to convey the meaning intended in this report.

Phenome-Wide Association Study (PheWAS) akin to the genome-wide association studies (GWAS) widely used today to find single nucleotide polymorphisms (SNPs) that are genetically linked in a population to a particular disease trait—except that PheWAS is GWAS in reverse. GWAS associates genotypes with a given phenotype, such as height or a genetic disease. In contrast, PheWAS attempts to determine the range of clinical phenotypes associated with a given genotype (Mak 2011).

Phenotype the idiosyncratic traits exhibited by an organism, often categorized in terms of known trait variants. This can either refer to a specific trait or to a collection of traits. For example, blue eyes and brown eyes are phenotypes exhibited in subsets of humans.

Phenotype-genotype association (or correlation) the association between the presence of a certain mutation or mutations (genotype) and the resulting physical trait, abnormality, or pattern of abnormalities (phenotype). With respect to genetic testing, the frequency with which a certain phenotype is observed in the presence of a specific genotype determines the positive predictive value of the test (http://ghr.nlm.nih.gov/glossary=genotypephenotypecorrelation).

Precision medicine (also see: Personalized Medicine) as used in this report, "precision medicine" refers to the tailoring of medical treatment to the individual characteristics of each patient. It does not literally mean the creation of drugs or medical devices that are unique to a patient, but rather the ability to classify individuals into subpopulations that differ in their susceptibility to a particular disease, in the biology and/or prognosis of those diseases they may develop, or in their response to a specific treatment. Preventive or therapeutic interventions can then be concentrated on those who will benefit, sparing expense and side effects for those who will not. Although the term "personalized medicine" is also used to convey this meaning, that term is sometimes misinterpreted as implying that unique treatments can be designed for each individual. For this reason, the Committee thinks that the term "precision medicine" is preferable to "personalized medicine" to convey the meaning intended in this report. It should be emphasized that in "precision medicine" the word "precision" is being used in a colloquial sense, to mean both "accurate" and "precise" (in the scientific method, the **accuracy** of a measurement system is the degree of closeness of measurements of a quantity to that quantity's actual (true) value whereas the **precision** of a measurement system, also called reproducibility or repeatability, is the degree to which repeated measurements under unchanged conditions show the same results). http://en.wikipedia.org/wiki/Accuracy_and_precision. the point where pharmacogenetics and personalised medicine meet (The Economist 2009).

Precompetitive collaboration collaboration among competitors to achieve goals that can be more effectively accomplished by a group effort and have the potential to benefit everyone (IOM 2010a).

Proteome the entire complement of proteins and associated modifications produced by an organism (PCAST 2008).

Public–private partnerships agreement between a public agency (federal, state, or local) and a private sector entity. Through this agreement, the skills and assets of each sector (public and private) are shared in delivering a service or facility for the use of the general public (NCPP 2011).

Radioisotopic labeling the incorporation of radioactive atoms into DNA so that the DNA can be detected and visualized based on its emission of radioactivity.

Recombinant DNA the artificial synthesis of sequences of DNA that may or may not exist in nature using genetic engineering techniques. These techniques are central to much of molecular biology and to the development of modern drugs.

Sequelae a pathological condition resulting from a prior disease, injury, or attack (MedicineNet.com. 2011).

Single Nucleotide Polymorphism (SNP) single genetic variation; DNA sequence variations caused by single base changes at a given position in a genome. (PCAST 2008).

Signs and symptoms objective evidence of disease perceptible to the examining physician (sign) and subjective evidence of disease perceived by the patient (symptom).

Social network an association of people drawn together by family, work, or hobby.

Systematized Nomenclature of Medicine (SNOMED) a comprehensive clinical terminology, originally created by the College of American Pathologists (CAP) and, as of April 2007, owned, maintained, and distributed by the International Health Terminology Standards Development Organisation (IHTSDO), a not-for-profit association in Denmark.

Systems analyses analysis of all aspects of a project along with ways to collect information about the operation of its parts (wordnetweb.princeton.edu/perl/webwn).

Transcriptome the complete set of RNA transcripts produced by the genome at any one time. The transcriptome is dynamic and changes under different circumstances due to different patterns of gene expression. The study of the transcriptome is termed transcriptomics (MedicineNet.com. 2011).

Translational research transforms scientific discoveries arising from laboratory, clinical, or population studies into clinical applications to reduce cancer incidence, morbidity, and mortality. (NCI 2011). http://www.cancer.gov/researchandfunding/trwg/TRWG-definition-and-TR-continuum.

Whole-genome sequencing determining the sequence of deoxyribonucleotides that compose an entire genome, including all of its chromosomes.

GLOSSARY REFERENCES

APOR (The Association for Patient Oriented Research). 2011 APOR http://www.apor.org/[accessed October 10, 2011].

Economist. 2009. Getting Personal: The Promise of Cheap Genome Sequencing. The Economist, April 16, 2009 [online]. Available: http://www.economist.com/node/13437974?story_id=13437974 [accessed September 13, 2011].

ESRI (Environmental Systems Research Institute, Inc.). 1990. In Understanding GIS: The ARC/INFO Method. Redlands, CA: ESRI, Pp. 1-2.

Garets, D., and M. Davis. 2005. Electronic Patient Records: EMRs and EHRs. Healthcare Informatics [online]. Available: http://www.providersedge.com/ehdocs/ehr_articles/Electronic_Patient_Records-EMRs_and_EHRs.pdf [accessed Aug. 25, 2011].

Hooper, L.V., and J.I. Gordon. 2001. Comensal host-bacterial relationships in the gut. Science 292(5519):1115-1118.

Houghton Mifflin Company. 2007. The American Heritage Medical Dictionary. Boston, MA: Houghton Mifflin Company.

InfoGlobalLink. 2011. Gene Expression Analysis [online]. Available: http://www.infogloballink.com/gene-sequencing/ [accessed September 13, 2011].

Information Buiders. 2011. Decision Support Systems-DSS [online]. Available: http://www.informationbuilders.com/decision-support-systems-dss [accessed Aug. 30, 2011].

IOM (Institute of Medicine). 2010a. Extending the Spectrum of Precompetitive Collaboration in Oncology Research: Workshop Summary. M. Patlack, S. Nass, E. Balogh, eds. Washington, DC: National Academies Press.

IOM (Institute of Medicine). 2010b. Microbial Evolution and Co-Adaptation. Washington, DC: National Academies Press.

Kahn, T.J., and H.S. Ninomiya, eds. 2010. Bioethics Thesaurus for Genetics. Washington, DC: Georgetown University [online]. Available: http://genethx.georgetown.edu/BioethicsThesaurusForGeneticsSearchersGuide.pdf [accessed October 10, 2011].

Khoury, M.J. 2003. Genetics and genomics in practice: The continuum from genetic disease to genetic information in health and disease. Genet. Med. 5(4):261-268).

Liddy, E.D. 2001. Natural language processing. In Encyclopedia of Library and Information Science, 2nd ed. New York: Marcel Decker [online]. Available: http://www.cnlp.org/publications/03NLP.LIS.Encyclopedia.pdf [accessed October 10, 2011].

Mak, H.C. 2011. Discovery from data repositories. Nat. Biotechnol. 29:46-47.

McGraw-Hill. 2002. Concise Dictionary of Modern Medicine. The McGraw-Hill Companies, Inc.

Medical Dictionary. 2011. Medical Dictionary [online]. Available: http://de.dict.md/definition/markers

MedicineNet.com. 2011. Medical Dictionary [online]. Available: http://www.medterms.com/script/main/hp.asp [accessed September 13, 2011].

Merriam-Webster. 2007.Merriam-Webster's Dictionary [online]. Available: http://www.merriam-webster.com/browse/dictionary/a.htm?&t=1314709194 [accessed Aug. 30, 2011]

Mizrachi, I. .2002. GenBank: The Nucleotide Sequence Database. Chapter 1 in the NCBI Handbook, J. McEntype, and J. Ostell, eds. Bethesda: National Center for Biotecnology Information.

Moore, G. 1965. Cramming more components onto integrated circuits. Electronics 38(8) [online]. Available:ftp://download.intel.com/museum/Moores_Law/Articles-Press_Releases/Gordon_Moore_1965_Article.pdf [accessed September 13, 2011].

Mosby. 2009. Mosby's Medical Dictionary, 8th ed. Elsevier.

NCBI (National Center for Biotechnology Information). 2011. dbGap: Database of Genotypes and Phenotypes. National Center for Biotechnology Information [online]. Available: http://www.ncbi.nlm.nih.gov/ [accessed Aug. 5, 2011].

NCI (National Cancer Institute). 2011. TRWG Definition of Translational Research [online]. Available: http://www.cancer.gov/researchandfunding/trwg/TRWG-definition-and-TR-continuum [accessed September 13, 2011].

NCPP (National Council for Public-Private Partnership). 2011. How PPPs Work [online]. Available: http://ncppp.org/howpart/index.shtml [accessed October 10, 2011].

NHGRI (National Human Genome Research Institute]. 2011. Talking Glossary of Genetics Terms [online]. Available: http://www.genome.gov/Glossary/index.cfm [accessed Aug. 25, 2011].

PCAST (President's Council of Advisors on Science and Technology). 2008. Priorities for Personalized Medicine. President's Council of Advisors on Science and Technology, September 2008 [online]. Available: http://www.whitehouse.gov/files/documents/ostp/PCAST/pcast_report_v2.pdf [accessed August 3, 2011].

Pigeot, I. 2005. Handbook of Epidemiology. Berlin: Springer, P. 95.

Quehenberger, O., A.M. Armando, A.H. Brown, S.B. Milne, D.S. Myers, A.H. Merrill, S. Bandyopadhyay, K.N. Jones, S. Kelly, R.L. Shaner, C.M. Sullards, E. Wang, R.C. Murphy, R.M. Barkley, T.J. Leiker, C.R. H. Raetz, Z. Guan, G.M. Laird, D.A. Six, D.W. Russell, J.G. McDonald, S. Subramaniam, E. Fahy, and E.A. Dennis. 2010. Lipidomics reveals a remarkable diversity of lipids in human plasma. J. Lipid Res. 51(11):3299-3305.

Rappaport, S.M. 2011. Implications of the exposome for exposure science. J. Expo. Sci. Environ. Epidemiol. 21(1):5-9.

Science Dictionary. 2011. Science Dictionary.com [online]. Available: http://www.science-dictionary.com/definition/epigenome.html [accessed October 10, 2011].

USC (University of South California). 2011. Glossary. University of South California Norris Comprehensive Cancer Center [online]. Available: http://uscnorriscancer.usc.edu/glossary/ [accessed Aug. 25, 2011].

Wild, C.P. 2005. Complementing the genome with an "exposome": The outstanding challenge of environmental exposure measurement in molecular epidemiology. Cancer Epidemiol. Biomarkers Prev. 14(8):1847-1850.

Wishar, D.S, D. Tzur, C. Knox, R. Eisner, A.C. Guo, N. Young, D. Cheng, K. Jewell, D. Arndt, S. Sawhney, C. Fung, L. Nikolai, M. Lewis, M.A. Coutouly, I. Forsythe, P. Tang, S. Shrivastava, K. Jeroncic, P. Stothard, G. Amegbey, D. Block, D.D. Hau, J. Wagner, J. Miniaci, M. Clements, M. Gebremedhin, N. Guo, Y. Zhang, G.E. Duggan, G.D. Macinnis, A.M. Weljie, R. Dowlatabadi, F. Bamforth, D. Clive, R. Greiner, L. Li, T. Marrie, B.D. Sykes, H.J. Vogel, and L. Querengesser. 2007. HMDB: The Human Metabolome Database. Nucleic Acids Res. 35:D521-D526.